NUTRITION
&
HEALTH

This new series is designed to meet the growing demand for current, accessible information about the increasingly popular wellness approach to personal health. The result of a collaborative effort by a highly professional writing, editorial, and publishing team, the *Wellness* series consists of 16 volumes, each on a single topic. Each volume in this attractively produced series combines original material with carefully selected readings, relevant statistical data, and illustrations. The series objectives are to increase awareness of the value of a wellness approach to personal health and to help the reader become a more informed consumer of health-related information. Employing a critical thinking approach, each volume includes a variety of assessment tools, discusses basic concepts, suggests key questions, and provides the reader with a list of resources for further exploration.

James K. Jackson	Wellness: AIDS, STD, & Other Communicable Diseases
Richard G. Schlaadt	Wellness: Alcohol Use & Abuse
Richard G. Schlaadt	Wellness: Drugs, Society, & Behavior
Robert E. Kime	Wellness: Environment & Health
Gary Klug & Janice Lettunich	Wellness: Exercise & Physical Fitness
James D. Porterfield & Richard St. Pierre	Wellness: Healthful Aging
Robert E. Kime	Wellness: The Informed Health Consumer
Paula F. Ciesielski	Wellness: Major Chronic Diseases
Robert E. Kime	Wellness: Mental Health
Judith S. Hurley	Wellness: Nutrition & Health
Robert E. Kime	Wellness: Pregnancy, Childbirth, & Parenting
David C. Lawson	Wellness: Safety & Accident Prevention
Randall R. Cottrell	Wellness: Stress Management
Richard G. Schlaadt	Wellness: Tobacco & Health
Randall R. Cottrell	Wellness: Weight Control
Judith S. Hurley & Richard G. Schlaadt	Wellness: The Wellness Life-Style

NUTRITION & HEALTH

Judith S. Hurley, M.S., R.D.

WELLNESS

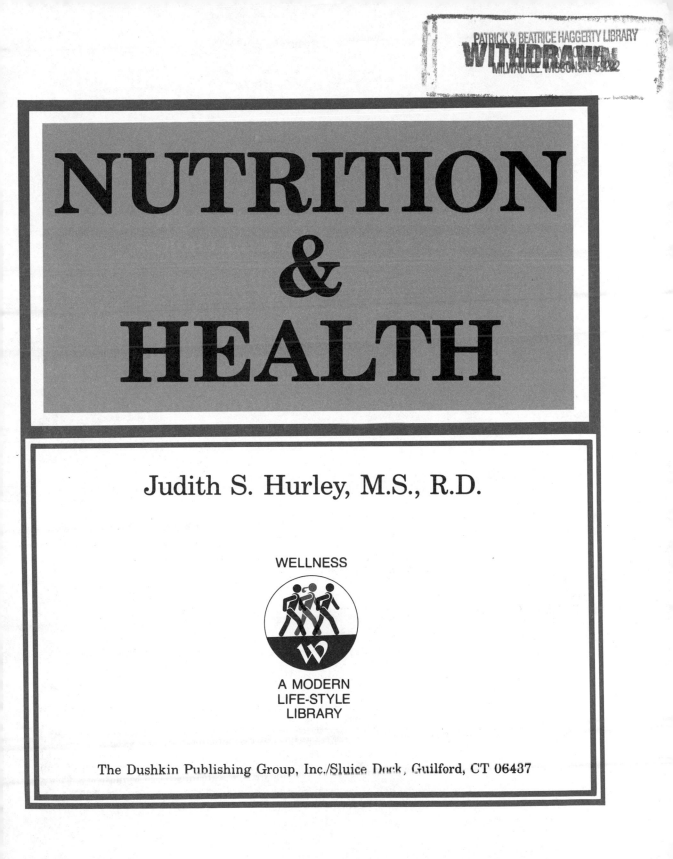

A MODERN
LIFE-STYLE
LIBRARY

The Dushkin Publishing Group, Inc./Sluice Dock, Guilford, CT 06437

To Samara, Melissa, and Dana

Library of Congress Catalog Card Number: 90-084121
Manufactured in the United States of America
First Edition, First Printing
ISBN: 0-87967-875-5

Library of Congress Cataloging-in-Publication Data

Hurley, Judith S., Nutrition & Health (Wellness)
    1. Nutrition. 2. Health. I. Title. II. Series.
TX364   613.2   90-084121   ISBN 0-87967-875-5

Please see page 178 for credits.

The procedures and explanations given in this publication are based on research and consultation with medical and nursing authorities. To the best of our knowledge, these procedures and explanations reflect currently accepted medical practice; nevertheless, they cannot be considered absolute and universal recommendations. For individual application, treatment suggestions must be considered in light of the individual's health, subject to a doctor's specific recommendations. The authors and the publisher disclaim responsibility for any adverse effects resulting directly or indirectly from the suggested procedures, from any undetected errors, or from the reader's misunderstanding of the text.

JUDITH S. HURLEY

Judith S. Hurley, M.S., R.D., is a nutrition and health consultant. She was formerly Director of Employee Health Promotion for New Mexico State Government, health consultant to Los Alamos National Laboratory, a clinical nutritionist, and an instructor of nutrition at the University of Oregon. She currently consults on an international nutrition project of the U.S. National Cancer Institute and provides health promotion planning, nutrition education, and employee wellness programs to government agencies and corporations.

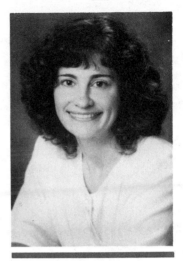

WELLNESS:
A Modern Life-Style Library

General Editors
Robert E. Kime, Ph.D.
Richard G. Schlaadt, Ed.D.

Authors
Paula F. Ciesielski, M.D.
Randall R. Cottrell, Ed.D.
Judith S. Hurley, M.S., R.D.
James K. Jackson, M.D.
Robert E. Kime, Ph.D.
Gary A. Klug, Ph.D.
David C. Lawson, Ph.D.
Janice Lettunich, M.S.
James D. Porterfield
Richard St. Pierre, Ph.D.
Richard G. Schlaadt, Ed.D.

Developmental Staff
Irving Rockwood, Program Manager
Paula Edelson, Series Editor
Carolyn Dickinson, Administrative Assistant
Jason J. Marchi, Editorial Assistant

Editing Staff
John S. L. Holland, Managing Editor
Marcuss Oslander, Editor
Diane Barker, Editorial Assistant
Mary L. Strieff, Art Editor
Robert Reynolds, Illustrator

Production and Design Staff
Brenda S. Filley, Production Manager
Whit Vye, Cover Design and Logo
Jeremiah B. Lighter, Text Design
Libra Ann Cusack, Typesetting Supervisor
Charles Vitelli, Designer
Meredith Scheld, Graphics Assistant
Steve Shumaker, Graphics Assistant
Juliana Arbo, Typesetter
Richard Tietjen, Editorial Systems Analyst

Preface

NO ONE WHO likes to eat as much as I do and who is as fascinated by the quirky and varied eating habits of our time as I am could resist the opportunity to write a book about nutrition.

During the span of time when this book was written, my own diet included fried guinea pig washed down with Coca Cola in the highlands of Ecuador; fresh snapper, sliced and eaten sashimi-style within minutes of being caught in a tropical sea; fast-food hamburgers served alongside the interstate; soyburgers served alongside brown rice; chicken baked with forty cloves of garlic; enchiladas smothered with fiery green chile; and one of the most surprisingly delicious things I have ever eaten, a bowl of wild greens in broth, graciously served up by a Mexican family who had, quite literally, nothing else in the larder. Thankfully, the wisdom of diverse cultures and the science of nutrition both teach the same thing—that the human body is tremendously adaptable and able to obtain its basic nutritional needs from an astonishing variety of foods and eating patterns.

Most people are quite confused these days by the topic of nutrition. As in other areas of health, experts disagree what is "good" for people. Among other things, nutritional scientists differ in their interpretations of research, their assessments of dietary risks and food safety issues, and their views of the proper role of government with respect to regulation of the food industry. Nonetheless, we now know enough to make responsible dietary recommendations, even though those recommendations may change as new information comes to light.

Wellness: Nutrition & Health will familiarize you with the current dietary guidelines for health and provide the tools you need to make appropriate changes in your diet. And in an age when typical eating habits can contribute to poor fitness, lack of energy, and development of heart disease, cancer, and other illnesses, the time to begin making those positive changes has arrived. A number of self-assessments and planning aids are included to help you develop better eating habits along with articles that explore up-to-the-minute nutritional concerns. The resources at the end of the book are excellent stepping stones to further exploration, if you are so inclined.

This is not a definitive work, but rather a place to begin. The central objective of this book is not to make you into an instant expert but to help you learn to *think critically* about the nutritional claims and counterclaims with which all of us are bombarded daily. Only then will you be able to distinguish nutritional fact from myth, and only then will you be an informed consumer.

The hundreds of students and nutrition program participants I have worked with through the years have contributed considerably to this book. Without their insights and questions, I would not know which topics concern, confuse, and worry people and which suggestions and information they find useful and realistically applicable in their lives. Most importantly, they have shown me why, in a field rife with controversies and a burgeoning marketplace of new food products, it is important to encourage critical thinking and decision-making rather than to present pat answers.

Several people very kindly contributed their expertise and assistance with the development of this book. I am indebted to Professor Roberta Hollander of Howard University and Janice Montgomery, R.D., for their careful review of the manuscript and many useful suggestions. In addition, Stephen Barrett, M.D., provided review and comment, and the general series editors, Dick Schlaadt and Bob Kime of University of Oregon, offered support and encouragement from the beginning. Carolyn Dickinson of The Dushkin Publishing Group competently and graciously took care of numerous last-minute details. And not least, I extend my thanks to Irving Rockwood, program manager at the DPG, who was unfailingly helpful throughout, providing welcomed guidance with wisdom, warmth, and humor.

Judith S. Hurley
Quito, Equador

Contents

1
Our Food Environment
Page 1

2
The Balancing Act
Page 22

3
Game Plan For A Healthy Diet
The Nutrients Energy Balance Carbohydrates
Page 46

5

Game Plan For A Healthy Diet

Water • Vitamins
Minerals
Page 106

6

Making Choices

Page 133

FIGURES

TABLES

Our Food Environment

"Tell me what you eat and I will tell you what you are."

Jean Anthelme Brillat-Savarin, philosopher and gastronome, 1825

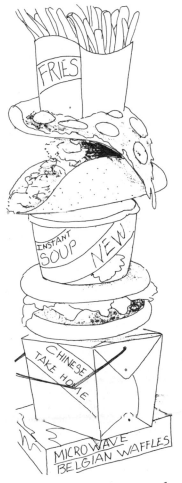

WE SHOUT OUR REQUEST into the microphone and drive forward to receive a little bag of food whose contents are identical to thousands of other little bags in cities throughout the country. At the supermarket, into our shopping cart go plastic bags, metal cans, aluminum pop-tops, cardboard cartons, flavor packets, bubble wraps, foil-sealed bags, vacuum-sealed bags, and other bright, flashy packages. They contain presliced, prebaked, preseasoned, irradiated, heat-processed, flash-frozen, chemically cured, scientifically preserved, artificially flavored, synthetically colored, fat-laden, salted, sugar-saturated food. Down the aisle are coffee and bananas from Central America, soy sauce from Japan, marmalades from England, kiwi fruit from New Zealand and melons from Mexico. Driving through any large city we see restaurants that serve Mexican food, Chinese food, Middle Eastern food, Italian food, and a host of other cuisines. Cookbooks, cooking videos, and cooking classes on foods of every corner of the world are available. Hungry? The solution for most people is as close as the vending machine down the hall, the corner doughnut shop, or the late night convenience store. More than any time in history we have available a multitude of foods, both nutritious and not-so-nutritious. And more than any time in history, we are faced with choices, choices, choices. . . .

Although granola cereals usually contain whole grains, most are also heavily sweetened and contain lots of fat in the form of nuts, oil, and coconut.

THE NEW AMERICAN DIET

Most average Americans will drink 40 gallons of soft drinks this year, consume nearly 40 teaspoons of sugar and 2 to 3 teaspoons of salt each day, take in 3 out of every 5 **calories** as fat and sugar, eat nearly half of their meals away from home, and consume half of their food in a processed rather than fresh form (1,2,3). Although they will consume fewer calories than their grandparents did at their age, they will more likely become overweight because of a less active lifestyle (1).

Food habits in the United States are quite different from those of even 50 years ago and this new American diet is contributing to the high incidence of heart disease, stroke, cancer, overweight, and hypertension seen in the United States and other industrialized countries.

TOO MANY CHOICES?

Available food choices and our food habits in the United States have changed so much during recent decades that many people have little concept of what constitutes a traditional, healthy diet or eating pattern. The old recommendations to "eat three square meals a day" or "follow the four food groups" no longer seem adequate to guide us through the maze of choices. Many healthy foods are available, but they are frequently outnumbered by the less nutritious, heavily promoted food products that appear at dizzying rates in our supermarkets and restaurants. And the easy access to this large array of foods means that poor choices are often more convenient to make than healthy ones. It is easy to take the course of least resistance and choose the quick and the familiar—all too often the fatty, the sweet, and the salty. In fact, the average American diet is now comprised of nearly 60 percent fat and sugar (4).

In addition, the many sources of nutrition information competing for our attention often provide confusing or contradictory information. Supermarket shelves offer some 15,000 different items, newspapers report on the latest research findings one week only to report contradictory findings the next, and advertisements from television, billboards, magazines, and food packages bombard us. To make matters more confusing, the current interest in nutrition has spawned a large market for products sold as health foods and super foods such as spirulina algae, wheat germ, fish oils, and protein powders. Like a bewildered

Calorie: Technically, a unit used to measure energy equivalent to the amount of heat that raises the temperature of 1 gram of water 1 degree centigrade. Calories in food represent the energy value of the food, and are measured in kilocalories (a thousand calories), although in common usage we refer to these kilocalories simply as calories.

(continued on p. 4)

Americans may know their food facts, but they still believe in quick fixes and cutting out, rather than cutting down, according to a recent Gallup Poll. The poll was commissioned by ADA* and the International Food Information Council (IFIC) and released in late February [1990]. "The survey findings point to a vital role for registered dietitians as food and nutrition experts who can help translate the science of nutrition into

How Americans Make Food Choices: Results of a Gallup Poll

healthy food choices," explains President Nancy S. Wellman, PhD, RD. Common-sense messages like those of National Nutrition Month® can help busy Americans increase their nutrition knowledge and make sound decisions about the foods they eat. The graph below illustrates some of the survey findings.

Although 95 percent of Americans believe balance, variety, and moderation are the keys to healthy eating, many fail to apply their nutrition IQ when selecting foods, according to the ADA-IFIC Gallup Poll. The survey results, announced at a New York press conference revealed that two-thirds of the public choose foods based on whether they perceive them to be "good" or "bad."

At the press conference, Wellman explained that "Americans are surprisingly knowledgeable about nutrition and health, but when it

*American Dietetic Association

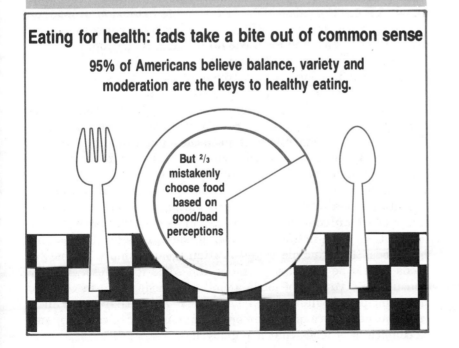

Eating for health: fads take a bite out of common sense

95% of Americans believe balance, variety and moderation are the keys to healthy eating.

But ²/₃ mistakenly choose food based on good/bad perceptions

Where's the Beef?
Ask a Teenager

The good news from a recent survey of home economics students (the Fifth Annual Teen Food and Nutrition survey) is that teens are increasingly aware of the importance of good nutrition. When asked about cholesterol, for example, some 36 percent of those surveyed said they are aware of what serum cholesterol means to their health.

The bad news is that this knowledge doesn't always translate into action. Although 48 percent indicated that awareness of cholesterol influences their food purchases, 43 percent expressed a preference for beef as a protein source and another 12 percent mentioned pork. Similarly, 74 percent said potato chips are their favorite snack food followed by ice cream (72 percent) and candy (68 percent).

comes to translating facts into food choices, most still opt for quick fixes and the latest health fads."

The nationally projectable survey involved 762 men and women aged 18 years and older. Among the inconsistencies highlighted by the survey:

- 50 percent of respondents said they are increasing their consumption of oat bran or vitamin supplements due to health concerns. But only 8 percent reported increasing consumption of fruits or fruit juices.
- 45 percent of survey respondents said they are eliminating red meat, while 36 percent are cutting out dairy foods due to health concerns. More women than men reported eliminating meat and dairy products totally, despite current advice to improve intake of iron and calcium from lowfat sources.
- 81 percent knew that blood cholesterol levels are affected by factors other than diet, such as heredity, high blood pressure, smoking and exercise. But 50 percent are still unaware of the difference between blood cholesterol and dietary cholesterol.

Source: *American Dietetic Association Courier*, Vol. 29, No. 3, March 1990, p. 2.

Nutrients: Compounds used by the body for growth, maintenance, and repair. Nutrients are essential to life and most cannot be manufactured by the body and must be taken in through food.

Alice in Wonderland, we are faced with new delectables urging "Eat me! Drink me!" Books on nutrition and diet abound, talk shows feature the latest diet doctor or life extension proponent and magazines are filled with diet regimens for runners, executives, vegetarians, and even the family dog. Nutrition, it seems, has become big business! Amidst all the babel, how does one sort out facts from fallacies, truths from half-truths, and determine an intelligent strategy for one's own eating habits?

In spite of all the debates, controversies, and recommendations that appear about everything from food additives to cholesterol to fiber, three basic principles still form the foundation for a healthy diet: variety, moderation, and balance. Different foods contain different **nutrients**. Eating a wide variety of foods is thus the first step in ensuring one takes in the nearly 50 nutrients essential to health. With so many tempting foods around us that make overindulgence easy, moderation becomes important. But rather than rigid notions about what constitutes good foods and bad foods, the principle of moderation means simply that some foods should be emphasized more and some foods less. And by consuming a variety of foods along with moderation in choices, the principle of balance can be achieved—a diet that meets one's nutrient needs, provides the appropriate number of calories, and is comprised of foods that are enjoyed.

(continued on p. 8)

Would You Take Diet Advice From an Overweight Expert?

And Other Questions From Our Gallup Poll

What's really going on out there? We're pouring a lot less whole milk but filling our bowls with ice cream. We're avoiding beef and pork, and digging into buckets of deep-fried chicken nuggets with the skin blended in. Esoteric "HDLs" and "LDLs" are threatening to become household terms, yet we still don't know the best way to lower our own cholesterol. At the same time, other messages *are* getting through: Not a single person who responded to this survey could be tricked into saying we're in danger of eating too much fiber.

Most of what we know about our changing and sometimes contradictory nutritional landscape is drawn from acres of statistics on what America is actually eating. This poll, however, is more concerned with what's in our heads than on our plates. It reveals some of our attitudes, in the supermarket and at the dinner table. What are we really worrying about? What do we think we should be trying to do with our diets? And just whose advice do we value?

Americans don't get the big nutrition message

"The Surgeon General recently singled out the chief health problem in the diets of Americans. He says our food contains too much. . . "

Cholesterol 48%
Fat 17%
Salt 11%
Pesticides 7%
Sugar...................................6%
Fiber 0%
Don't know..............................11%

This is the big test on the *one* thing all Americans ought to know about smart eating. And we flunked. Not even one in five Americans knows what substance the Surgeon General actually slammed—fat, not cholesterol, as nearly half of us think. Fat, he pointed out, is the one sub-

stance in our food that's been implicated in both heart disease and cancer.

We don't know the best way to lower our cholesterol

"If you learned that you have a high blood cholesterol level that puts you at risk of heart disease, which would you say is the single most important dietary change you should make? Would you eat foods. . . "

Lower in cholesterol 36%
Higher in fiber 26%
Lower in saturated fat.................18%
Lower in fat...........................17%
Don't know 3%

More than a third of Americans mistakenly think cholesterol-counting is the best way to lower blood cholesterol, and about a quarter would look for foods high in fiber. Not many have grasped health experts' message that saturated fat—not dietary cholesterol—has the greatest effect in raising cholesterol. Researchers don't know the exact mechanisms, but plenty of studies have shown that while dietary cholesterol can raise blood cholesterol, saturated fat has an even stronger effect. It doesn't seem to make sense—which is probably why many Americans have such odd diets: They'll trade eggs for oat bran cereal, then have double scoops of ice cream later in the day.

People who've attended college are more than twice as likely to avoid saturated fat as those who haven't finished high school (24 percent to 10). Seatbelt users also correctly chose saturated fat more often than did nonusers (20 percent to 12).

We take scary food news seriously

"When you learn that a certain food is high in a substance linked to cancer or heart disease, what is your usual reaction?"

Just eat less of that food..............46%
Stop eating that food altogether.......26%
Ignore the news because it seems like
    everything causes some disease these
    days 21%
Ignore the news because I think
    researchers will just reverse their advice
    next year.............................6%
Don't know..............................1%

Almost three-fourths of us will start cutting back on a foodstuff as soon as we learn it's been linked to a health risk. Given all the alarms about cholesterol in meat and eggs, it's no wonder that Americans are eating less of them. We seem to be better at dodging specific foods than we are at following general advice, such as "Reduce your intake of saturated fat."

Health-conscious Americans—those who don't smoke, who exercise regularly, and who wear seatbelts—are more likely than smoking sedentary risktakers to completely give up worrisome foods (30 percent to 20). The risk-takers are much more comfortable ignoring food warnings because "It seems like everything causes some disease these days" (31 percent to 14).

We don't want the experts to choose "good" products for us

"The American Heart Association is planning to put its seal of approval on specific supermarket products that have healthful amounts of fat, cholesterol, and salt. Which statement comes closest to your point of view?"

I would prefer that the manufacturers give
    complete nutritional breakdowns and let
    me decide for myself...............43%
I would rather buy foods that have been
    labeled as healthful than have to figure
    out the right balance by myself.....35%
I already know enough about nutrition to
    make sensible choices..............18%
If health groups get away with this,
    supermarkets may stop offering the
    foods I like.........................3%
Don't know..............................1%

Almost two-thirds of Americans don't think the Heart Association's proposed seal of approval would be an appropriate or useful signpost to healthful products in supermarkets. The majority would rather do it themselves, with many preferring the manufacturer's help.

We think healthier food won't taste as good

"When you decide you want to make a change in your eating habits, but can't seem to do it, what would you say is the principal reason you usually don't make any changes?"

I don't think the food will taste
    as good 27%
I guess it's really not that important
    to me...............................22%
I don't have the time.................20%
I don't know how......................15%
Don't know 16%

We still seem to think meals that are good for us must be dull and flavorless, and it's evidently that perception—even more than apathy, lack of time, or ignorance—that's keeping Americans from making the eating changes they know they should.

We'd cut back on nutritious milk and meat before giving up dessert

"Medical researchers say you can lower your chances of heart disease by lowering fat in your diet. Which statement best describes your willingness to give up certain foods for possible long-term health benefits?"

I'm willing to eat half as much meat and
    whole milk dairy products 32%
I'm willing to give up potato chips and
    other junk food.....................30%
I'm willing to give up cheesecake and
    other rich desserts 16%
I'm willing to cut out all meat and whole
    milk dairy products.................14%
Until they can tell me how many more
    years I will live, I'm just going to eat
    what I like.........................10%
Don't know 4%*

To ditch some fat, Americans would much rather cut back on simple staples than give up rich desserts. It sounds bad, but there's a ray of hope: We're not nearly so attached to potato chips and related junk foods. When the third who'd give up junk foods are lumped in with the third who'd cut back on whole milk and meat, a trend appears: Given the right information, almost two-thirds of us would willingly take steps toward a healthier life. Vegetarianism is an option for almost one in six.

Those who smoke, spurn seatbelts, and don't get regular exercise are twice as likely as health-conscious respondents to say they'd eat whatever they like (16 percent to 8).

We think we're undernourished

"When it comes to vitamin and mineral supplements, which of the following statements best describes you?"

I'm not sure I get all the nutrients I need, but I do try to eat a variety of foods, so I don't take vitamin and mineral supplements 34%
I'm not sure I get all the nutrients I need, so I take multiple vitamins and mineral supplements daily 29%
I feel that I'm deficient in some nutrients, so I take specific vitamin and mineral supplements to compensate 13%
I already get all the nutrients I need, so I don't take vitamin and mineral supplements 12%
My doctor told me I'm deficient in some nutrients, so I take specific vitamin and mineral supplements to compensate 10%
Don't know 2%

Four out of five Americans believe they're coming up short on vitamins and minerals. To meet that concern, more than half of us are taking supplements—mostly without a health expert's recommendation. Another third are simply hoping to catch their nutrients in the mealtime cross-fire. Only 12 percent of us feel confident that we've gotten all the vitamins and minerals we need.

Almost half of us wouldn't trust an overweight health expert

"If you got diet or health advice from a doctor, nurse, or dietitian who was visibly overweight, what would be your reaction?"

I would just take the advice 54%
I would probably take the advice less seriously 30%
I would be inclined to ignore the advice 15%
Don't know 1%

The majority of Americans would simply take the word of overweight health experts, but then more than a quarter of Americans are overweight themselves. More remarkably, 45 percent of us think a fat expert isn't as trustworthy as a thin one—recognizing, perhaps, that extra weight has been linked to heart disease and other health risks.

Women are more likely than men (59 percent to 48) to say they would overlook the weight and just take the advice. Men, on the other hand, are marginally more likely to say they'd take the advice less seriously (33 percent to 28).

We'd pay extra for pesticide-free fruits and vegetables

"If you were offered a choice between ordinary supermarket produce and produce tested to show that it contains no pesticide residue, which statement best describes what you would buy?"

The tested produce, even if it costs a few cents more per pound 51%
The tested produce, even if it costs twice as much 25%
Whichever produce looks best, as long as it is the same price 21%
Don't know 3%

We're clearly worried that pesticide residues may be endangering our health. Three-quarters of Americans would pay more for fruits and vegetables shown to be free of pesticide residues, and many would pay *twice* as much—despite medical researchers' frequent assertions that there's no cause for concern.

Shoppers—who were found to be women by almost two to one—are more likely than non-shoppers to say they'd pay double for pristine fruits and vegetables (28 percent to 19). Those who aren't the household shoppers are more likely to say they'd buy whatever produce looked best (29 percent to 18).

We're no longer a "meat and potatoes" nation

"Which term comes closest to characterizing the type of food you typically eat for your day's main meal?"

Meat and potatoes .... .35%
Chicken and broccoli .... .34%
Brown rice and vegetables .... .12%
Pasta and salad .... .10%
Burger and fries. 5%
Pizza and soda. 3%
Don't know. 1%

"Real" people may drop their steak knives, but chicken and broccoli is now right up there with meat and potatoes as the handle for the classic American meal. And in third and fourth places are mountains of carbohydrates and vegetables. It's the greening of America—in self-image, at least.

Men are more likely than women (41 percent to 30) to peg themselves as meat-and-potato eaters. Sure enough, women are more likely than men to go for chicken and broccoli (40 percent to 27). Smokers and others who aren't taking extra steps to defend their health are much more likely than health-conscious Americans to pick meat and potatoes (45 percent to 26), while the health-conscious choose chicken and broccoli (40 percent to 25).

Source: *Hippocrates,* Vol. 3, No. 3, May/June 1989, pp. 46–48.

Moving towards a healthier diet also involves gaining knowledge about nutrition, observing current eating patterns, and learning to make appropriate changes. By understanding what is in the foods we choose and how different foods affect us, we can initiate changes in our eating pattern that may impact on our energy level, mood, physical stamina, and risk for several diseases. By making these changes enjoyably and gradually rather than all at once, we can make lasting improvements in our well-being.

MORE THAN NUTRIENTS

Our body cells and tissues must function, for better or for worse, with the food we take in as the source of energy and material needed for growth and repair. In this sense, our bodies can only be as healthy as the food we eat and the nutrients the food contains.

But food is more than just nutrients. We select foods for many reasons besides their health benefits. As one of the great pleasures of life, food occupies a central place in the special occasions, celebrations, and daily lives of people in all societies. Whether sitting down to an elaborate Thanksgiving dinner with family, going out for pizza with friends, enjoying a quiet breakfast alone, or putting on a pot of tea when someone drops by, we use food as a channel for companionship, sharing, and sensual delight as well as for appeasing our hunger and promoting our health. Special feasts, shared daily meals, and traditional foods give us a welcome sense of familiarity, belonging, and pleasure, and are an irreplaceable facet of our individual well-being and that of our families and communities. By selecting nutritious foods most of the time we can improve how we feel and our level of health and fitness—both important goals—but the other aspects of food justifiably guide our choices as well. Food nourishes us in many ways beyond supplying vitamins, minerals and other nutrients.

THE AMERICAN DIET IN TRANSITION

Is it any harder to be well-nourished now than in the past? The answer turns out not to be simple. With our well-developed system of food distribution we can buy a wider variety of foods than ever before all through the year. We also have access to more snack foods, high fat, and sugary foods. No longer reserved for special occasions or infrequent treats, they are available every day. In spite of this fact, one still needs as many nutrients as ever, provided in the right balance, to keep the body functioning at peak performance.

A look at the changes in the American diet during the last century reveals interesting trends. Foods provide us calories or energy in the form of protein, carbohydrate (starch and sugar), and fat. In 1910, only 32 percent of the calories in the American diet came from fat. Fat now provides approximately 37 percent of calories (5). Consumption of healthy **complex carbohydrate** foods (starches) has plummeted from 37 percent to only 21 percent of calories (5). At the same time, the amount of refined sugar and other sweeteners in the diet has increased from the 12 percent of calories consumed in 1910 to the current 18 percent (5). Why does the current American diet contain so much fat and sugar? Both the quantity of certain foods we eat and the preparation method are part of the answer.

Since 1910, fresh fruit consumption has decreased while intake of canned and frozen fruit, which often contains added sugar, has tripled (6). We are eating slightly more vegetables, but the increase is primarily in processed forms which are higher than fresh vegetables in sodium and sometimes fat. For example,

Complex carbohydrate: A polysaccharide, or compound consisting of many sugar molecules linked together. Complex carbohydrates in the diet include starches and the fiber, cellulose.

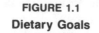

FIGURE 1.1
Dietary Goals

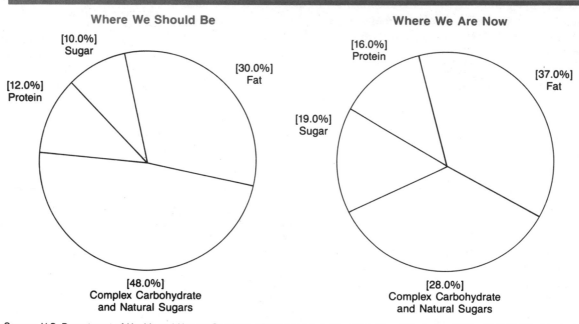

Source: U.S. Department of Health and Human Services, "Eating to Lower Your High Blood Cholesterol," No. 89-2920 (Washington, DC: Public Health Service, National Institute of Health, 1989).

According to the United States Department of Agriculture, approximately 37 percent of calories in the average American diet now comes from fat and 19 percent from sugar. In contrast, the United States' Dietary Goals call for a diet in which only 30 percent of the calories come from fat and 10 percent from sugar.

although we are eating more potatoes, the largest portion is now in the form of french fries and potato chips, providing us with a hefty dose of fat (6).

Total milk consumption has decreased, although people who do drink it are choosing whole milk less and low-fat and nonfat milk more (6). While intake of milk has gone down, consumption of soft drinks, with their often high sugar content (as much as 9 teaspoons in a 12-ounce can), has skyrocketed. Soft drink sales increased an explosive 600 percent between 1960 and 1975 to become a $10 billion per year business (7). In the United States, an average of 620 eight-ounce servings was consumed per person in 1980, over 3 times more than in 1960, and consumption has continued to rise in recent years (6).

We are eating a little less red meat today than in previous decades, but consumption is still higher than earlier in the century and provides approximately one-third of our fat intake (8). Cheese consumption has also increased, adding more fat to the diet (6).

FIGURE 1.2
Milk Consumption per Capita

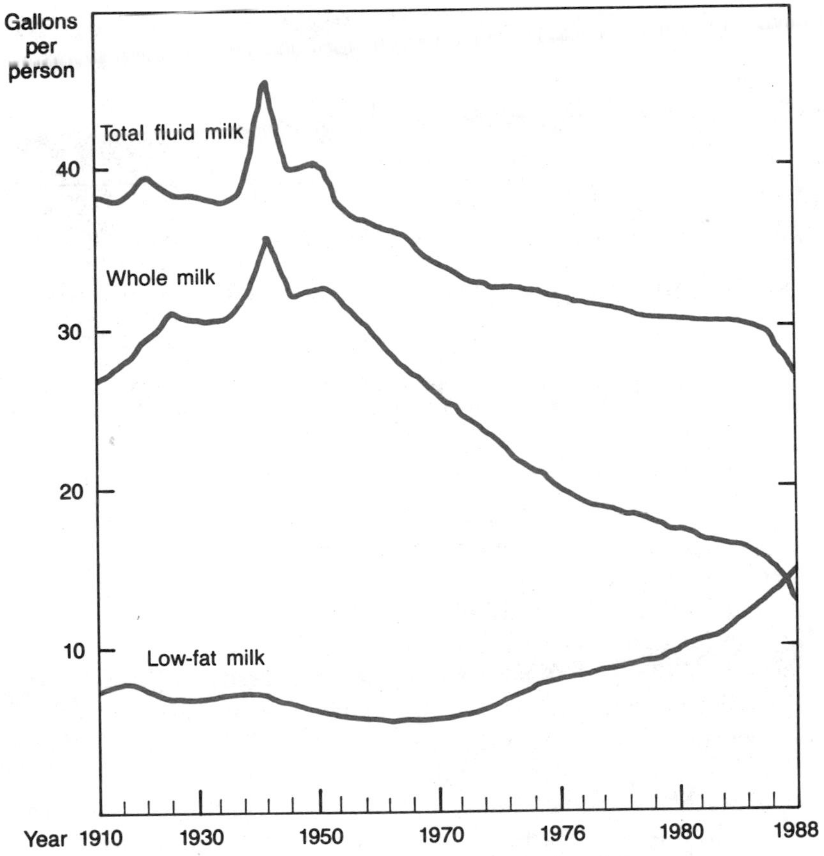

Source: United States Department of Agriculture.

Per capita consumption of whole milk has decreased dramatically in recent years while consumption of low-fat milk has increased. Overall, annual milk consumption has declined from approximately 38 gallons per capita in 1910 to approximately 26 gallons per capita in 1988.

Did You Know That . . .

Americans are eating eight times more broccoli today than they did 20 years ago. One result is that they're now getting eight times as much beta-carotene, vitamin C, calcium, and fiber from this nutrient-rich source than they were in 1970.

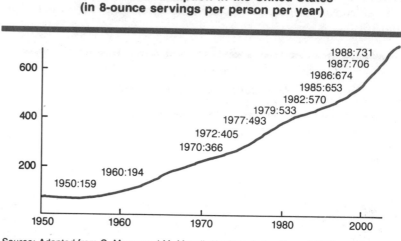

FIGURE 1.3

**Soft Drink Consumption in the United States
(in 8-ounce servings per person per year)**

1988:731
1987:706
1986:674
1985:653
1982:570
1979:533
1977:493
1972:405
1970:366
1960:194
1950:159

Source: Adapted from G. Moyer and M. Mayell, *Nutrition Action* (August 1981), p. 8, and *U.S. Industrial Outlook 1990*, pp. 34:26–29.

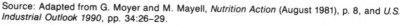

While milk consumption has decreased in recent decades, the consumption of soft drinks has skyrocketed. The average American now consumes more than 40 gallons of soft drinks yearly, which provide about 8 percent of the calories consumed daily. Such drinks have a very high sugar content. Each 12-ounce can of a typical cola drink, for example, contains approximately 9.2 teaspoons of sugar.

One of the most significant dietary changes since 1910 has been the decreased consumption of flours and grains, ideally a major part of a nutritious diet. We eat less than half the quantity of cereal products consumed in 1910 and have replaced it with foods high in fat and sugar (6).

Some of these changes correspond to transitions in our lifestyle. With increasingly fast-paced schedules for many, breakfast has become a hit-or-miss affair and is often skipped entirely. Once a tradition, only 25 percent of families eat breakfast together now (9). When breakfast is consumed, it may leave much to be desired. Many children's presweetened breakfast cereals contain over 50 percent sugar, providing even more sugar than a candy bar. And lunches are often haphazard. One recent poll reports over half of women aged 20 to 54 are dieting (10). Lunch is likely to be a salad or yogurt and little else. With both parents working in half the families in the United States, home-prepared meals are scarcer, and heat-and-serve convenience foods are relied on more heavily—often high in fat, salt, and sugar.

(continued on p. 17)

The Changing American Diet

If the United States got a Food Report Card, it would barely be pulling a C+ average. The Surgeon General and our other "teachers" have told us to eat:

- fewer fatty foods like red meat, cheese, whole milk, butter, and margarine,
- more complex carbohydrates like fruits, vegetables, whole grains, and beans, and
- fewer sugary foods like soft drinks, candy, and ice cream.

New figures from the U.S. Department of Agriculture show that we're following *some* of this advice. We're eating fewer eggs, less whole milk, and less beef than we did a decade ago. And avoiding the saturated fat and cholesterol in these foods has paid off. Since 1978, the number of Americans dying of heart disease has dropped by 29 percent.

But other changes show that we're not quite ready for the Honor Roll. Instead of replacing saturated fats with complex carbohydrates, we've replaced them with unsaturated fats.

"It's clear we haven't made much progress in getting people to eat less [total] fat, but we have been successful in changing the composition of fat," says Mark Hegsted, of Harvard University.

In other words, we're eating more chicken instead of beef, but it's fried chicken; more baked goods, but they're fatty baked goods; and more salads, but they're smothered in oily dressings.

It's not just our fat tooth that's insatiable. Despite the popularity of artificial sweeteners, we're consuming more sugars than ever before. And we now down more soft drinks than milk.

The influence of fast-food restaurants on our eating habits continues to grow. Chicken, soft drinks, salad, American and pizza cheese—just about all the foods we're eating more of are prominent on fast-food menus.

These grades rate not *what we eat*, but *how we've changed* what we eat over the last decade. For example, even though we still eat too many eggs (yolks), they get an "A," because we're eating fewer of them.

—Bonnie Liebman

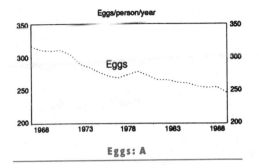

Eggs/person/year

Eggs: A

Egg-eating continues its 45-year decline, hitting a low of 234 per person in 1989. The cholesterol in the yolks is largely responsible, but it's only fair to acknowledge another reason: Moms who once had time to poach, boil, fry, or scramble are now scrambling to get to work.

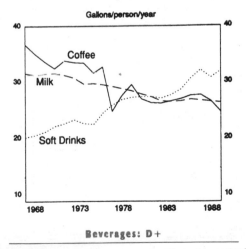

Gallons/person/year

Beverages: D+

Soft drinks have now surpassed milk as the nation's most popular beverage. And with milk consumption falling, the only reason Beverages didn't get an F is coffee's continuing 26-year decline. That's probably due to competition from soft drinks, concern about caffeine, quicker breakfasts, and central heating.

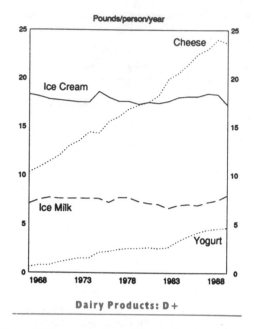

Dairy Products: D+

Since 1968, consumption of high-fat hard cheese has more than doubled. The reason? Fast-food pizzas and cheeseburgers. Yogurt's popularity continues to grow, in part because of its healthy reputation (which is well-deserved if it's low- or nonfat).

What's remarkable about our consumption of ice milk and ice cream is how little they've budged—either up or down.

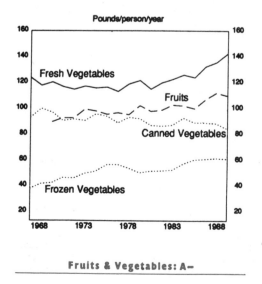

Fruits & Vegetables: A—

Potatoes, which account for about 37 percent of all fresh vegetables, and lettuce, which makes up about 17 percent, are both on the upswing, as are less-popular vegetables like broccoli, tomatoes, carrots, and cauliflower. We should probably thank fast-food baked potatoes and salad bars for both trends.

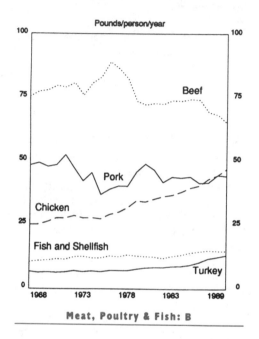

Meat, Poultry & Fish: B

No wonder the beef industry is running scared. Whether it's price or concern about clogged arteries, something seems to be curbing our taste for burgers, roasts, and steaks. All told, we ate 10 pounds less per person per year in the 1980s than the 1970s. Nevertheless, we still eat more beef than any other food in this group.

Why did we eat as much pork in the 1980s as in the 70s? Perhaps the industry's misleading ads, which call pork "The Other White Meat," have tricked us into thinking that pork is as low in fat as chicken, turkey, or fish (it isn't).

Chicken's rise isn't as promising as it seems. Most of the increase probably ends up as greasy nuggets, entrees, and McChicken sandwiches.

Turkey is finally breaking its Thanksgiving-Day stereotype, probably because it's being sold ground-up and in parts. Fish and shellfish consumption is only inching upwards, perhaps because prices have risen sharply. But much of the additional fish is fried fast-food, which is a far cry from broiled flounder.

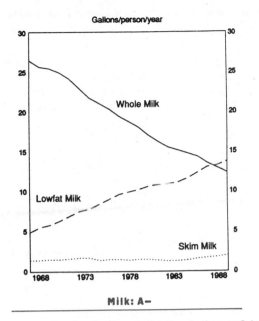

Milk: A–

Is the national milk glass half-full or half-empty? In 1960, lowfat milk was virtually non-existent. Now it has surpassed whole milk (terrific). But most of that "low-fat" is not-so-low two-percent milk, rather than truly-low one-percent (oops).

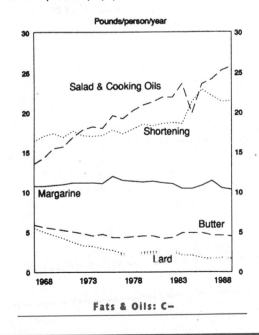

Fats & Oils: C–

We're eating 17 percent more complex carbohydrates than we did a decade ago (Yay!). That's largely due to a rise in wheat flour and rice. But we still eat less than half as much bread, cereal, pasta, and rice as our grandparents did in 1910.

The trick is to eat the bun without the burger, the pasta without the pesto, and the rice without the "roni."

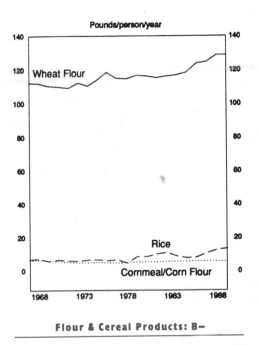

Flour & Cereal Products: B–

You might expect us to use less calorie-containing sweeteners like sugar or corn syrup as we eat more artificial ones. Wrong. Far from curbing the American sweet tooth, the switch has actually fed it. Apparently, the more we get, the more we want.

The charts overestimate what people actually eat, because they don't account for the food that gets thrown away . . . before or after it reaches our plates. Nevertheless, the figures are computed the same way for each food and for each year, so comparisons and changes are reliable.

Source: *Nutrition Action Healthletter,* Vol. 17, No. 4, May 1990, pp. 8, 9.

Noshing in the 90's: News of the Future

Fueled by growing health concerns and emerging technologies, the [current] decade promises to bring with it a plethora of new food products—and perhaps a new style of eating. Here's a crystal ball peek at the high-tech world of food that's on the way.

Nonfattening Fat. Imagine savoring bowls of creamy, guilt-free ice cream or chomping on chips fried in an oil without calories. This dieter's dream could come true with the approval of several new fat substitutes now under government scrutiny.

Two leaders of the pack are *Simplesse* (NutraSweet Co.) and olestra (Procter & Gamble). But other companies including Kraft General Foods, Frito-Lay and CPC International, makers of Best Foods, are hoping to introduce similar calorie-free or calorie-reduced fat substitutes.

Once approved, these new ingredients could crop up in ice cream, sour cream, cheeses, salad dressings, mayonnaise, dips and spreads. They may also replace old-fashioned fats for frying and baking.

What's the catch? No one really knows yet. Not everyone is convinced of the safety of these new products. And some question their value in promoting healthful habits or helping people lose weight. But other experts see a more promising future for fat substitutes. As more and more uses are approved, some predict fat substitutes could significantly slash the overall fat content of the average American's diet.

Calorie-Free Sugar. Though sugar substitutes may seem like yesterday's news, there could soon be an exciting new headliner. Unlike other artificial sweeteners such as saccharin, aspartame (*NutraSweet*) and the more recent acesulfame-K (*Sunette*), this future sugar is the real stuff . . . but it's totally calorie-free.

Referred to as a left-handed sugar (or L-sugar) because its molecular structure mirrors that of real sugar, this new-age sweetener called Lev-O-Cal, 'fools' the digestive tract and it goes unnoticed.

Supposedly, Lev-O-Cal looks and tastes like ordinary sugar, and because it has the same bulk as real sugar, it's usable in baking and cooking, an area where artificial sweeteners usually fall short.

Manufactured by Biospherics Corp. in Maryland, this yet-to-be approved sweetener holds high hopes for some. But other observers cite the absence of studies showing that low-calorie sweeteners are effective as long-term weight-loss aids. And critics complain that as the use of these sugar substitutes rises, obesity and sugar consumption actually increase. Nonetheless, since consumers aren't expected to outgrow their sweet tooth any time soon, manufacturers are continuing their search for the perfect replacement for sugar.

Other sweeteners that may reach the market in the future include alitame, sucralose, thaumatin, stevioside, and dihydrochalcones.

Designer Foods. Scores of food companies are currently dabbling in genetically-improved foods, according to the International Food Biotechnology Council in Washington, D.C. The organization has recently developed criteria and guidelines for evaluating the safety of such biotech foods.

So what's coming down the pike? Expect to see fruits and vegetables that are nutrient-enhanced, intensely flavored, and more resistant to pests and spoilage. All this accomplished by juggling the plant's genes.

Look for super carrots with 3 to 5 times as much beta carotene (vitamin A), crunchier carrot and celery snacks called VegiSnax, beta carotene-rich yellow cauliflower that 'looks like it was cooked in cheese sauce,' seed oils with a boost in monounsaturates, butter-flavored popcorn kernels, and decaffeinated coffee beans straight from the bush.

Through changes in breeding and feeding, we'll continue to see beef and pork that contains less fat. Experimental breeding of dairy cows and a change in their diets will help reduce the percentage of butterfat in milk before it's even bottled.

Tailor-Made Meals. "Prevention" will take on a new meaning as foods are tailor-made according to an individual's genetic make-up. Manufacturers will be marketing special foods to consumers who have genes predisposing them to heart disease, salt-sensitive hypertension, cancer or obesity.

Organically Grown Foods. The demand for organic foods will continue to grow. Consumers in the 80's became hypersensitive to the issue of pesticides on produce. Though many say the scare is unwarranted and pesticides pose little threat, grocers will be providing more certified-organic fruits and vegetables. The cost will be two to three times that of conventionally grown produce.

With the absence of a federal standard for "organic" produce, the guarantee of a truly chemical-free product may be difficult to come by. But consumer pressure may force a change, and stores may begin to employ their own inspectors.

Medicinal Foods. Health claims for food will reach an all-time high. Food companies in the 80's learned that nutrition sells, and in the 90's they will intensify their efforts to pitch products linked with particular health benefits—such as lowering blood cholesterol or fighting cancer.

This means manufacturers will continue to remove certain ingredients (like highly saturated tropical oils, cholesterol and sodium) and put in others (such as 'good fats' and fiber).

We've recently seen two major food manufacturers add to their cereals a high-fiber grain called psyllium—the main ingredient in certain over-the-counter laxatives, that have been found to lower blood cholesterol. A stir was created when, as a result, it caused the strict line between food and drugs to begin to blur. Some food futurists wonder where this will end.

The future of medicinal foods may be more clearly predicted when the Food and Drug Administration (FDA) completes drafting new regulations on health claims. These will fill a void created two years ago when the government lifted a long-standing ban against them.

As we look ahead to the nineties, there is a fork in the road. In one direction lies a return to nature via organic farming; in the other, an ever expanding universe of high tech foods. Whichever road we take, there are sure to be new ideas about diet and health, new discoveries about nutrients and amended dietary recommendations. But whatever happens, the next decade promises to be every bit as exciting as the one [we have left] behind.

—*Janet Helm, R.D.*

Source: *Environmental Nutrition,* December 1989.

Eating meals at restaurants has become a way of life, too. Thirty-nine cents out of every food dollar are spent in restaurants, and fast-food restaurants account for over 25 percent of our away-from-home meals (11).

Some nutritionists point out we have become a nation of grazers, continually foraging on bits of this and that throughout the day. This way of eating can be healthy given wise food choices. But a familiar scenario looks like this: forgoing breakfast, or quickly eating a piece of toast with juice, we nibble and snack our way through the morning on pastries and coffee, grab a hot dog or taco as we run lunch errands, and visit the vending machine for a mid-afternoon pick-me-up. Dinner is takeout from the local deli or a drive through a nearby fast-food outlet, and still unsatisfied, we sit in front of the TV and snack our way to bedtime.

These recent changes in eating patterns and available foods have advantages as well as disadvantages. Many more ethnic and foreign foods are now available and popular, adding immensely to the variety of choice. The trend toward high-fat gourmet cooking is paralleled by the move towards fresh, natural foods prepared with health as well as taste in mind. And restaurants have begun to respond to consumers' desires for healthy, low-fat dishes. With so many options available, we have only to apply a few basic principles of nutritional wisdom to develop a diet that is delicious and healthy. W

Eating Smart Quiz

Oils & Fats		Points
butter, margarine, shortening, mayonnaise, sour cream, lard, oil, salad dressing	I always add these to foods in cooking and/or at the table. 0	
	I occasionally add these to foods in cooking and/or at the table. 1	☐
	I rarely add these to foods in cooking and/or at the table. 2	
	I eat fried foods 3 or more times a week. 0	
	I eat fried foods 1-2 times a week. 1	☐
	I rarely eat fried foods. 2	

Dairy Products		
	I drink whole milk. 0	
	I drink 1%–2% fat-free milk. 1	☐
	I seldom eat frozen desserts or ice cream. 2	
	I eat ice cream almost every day. 0	
	Instead of ice cream, I eat ice milk, low-fat frozen yogurt & sherbet. 1	☐
	I eat only fruit ices, seldom eat frozen dairy dessert. 2	

Dairy Products (cont.)

	I eat mostly high-fat cheese (jack, cheddar, colby, Swiss, cream).	**0**	
	I eat both low and high-fat cheeses.	**1**	
	I eat mostly low-fat cheeses (pot, 2% cottage, skim milk mozzarella).	**2**	

Snacks

potato/corn chips, nuts, buttered popcorn, candy bars	I eat these every day.	**0**	
	I eat some occasionally.	**1**	
	I seldom or never eat these snacks.	**2**	

Baked Goods

pies, cakes, cookies, sweet rolls, doughnuts	I eat them 5 or more times a week.	**0**	
	I eat them 2–4 times a week.	**1**	
	I seldom eat baked goods or eat only low-fat baked goods.	**2**	

Poultry & Fish*

	I rarely eat these foods.	**0**	
	I eat them 1–2 times a week.	**1**	
	I eat them 3 or more times a week.	**2**	

Low-Fat Meats*

extra lean hamburger, round steak, pork loin roast, tenderloin, chuck roast	I rarely eat these foods.	**0**	
	I eat these foods occasionally.	**1**	
	I eat mostly fat-trimmed red meats.	**2**	

High-Fat Meat*

luncheon meats, bacon, hot dogs, sausage, steak, regular & lean ground beef	I eat these every day.	**0**	
	I eat these foods occasionally.	**1**	
	I rarely eat these foods.	**2**	

Cured & Smoked Meat & Fish*

luncheon meats, hot dogs, bacon, ham & other smoked or pickled meats and fish	I eat these foods 4 or more times a week.	0	
	I eat some 1–3 times a week.	1	
	I seldom eat these foods.	2	

Legumes

dried beans & peas: kidney, navy, lima, pinto, garbanzo, split-pea, lentil	I eat legumes less than once a week.	0	
	I eat these foods 1–2 times a week.	1	
	I eat them 3 or more times a week.	2	

Whole Grains & Cereals

whole grain breads, brown rice, pasta, whole grain cereals	I seldom eat such foods.	0	
	I eat them 2–3 times a day.	1	
	I eat them 4 or more times daily.	2	

Vitamin C-Rich Fruits & Vegetables

citrus fruits and juices, green pepper, strawberries, tomatoes	I seldom eat them.	0	
	I eat them 3–5 times a week.	1	
	I eat them 1–2 times a day.	2	

Dark Green & Deep Yellow Fruits & Vegetables**

broccoli, greens, carrots, peaches	I seldom eat them.	0	
	I eat them 3–5 times a week.	1	
	I eat them daily.	2	

Vegetables of the Cabbage Family

broccoli, cabbage, brussels sprouts, cauliflower	I seldom eat them.	0	
	I eat them 1–2 times a week.	1	
	I eat them 3–4 times a week.	2	

Alcohol

	I drink more than 2 oz. daily.	0	
	I drink alcohol every week but not daily.	1	
	I occasionally or never drink alcohol.	2	

Personal Weight

I'm more than 20 lbs. over my ideal weight.	0	
I'm 10–20 lbs. over my ideal weight.	1	☐
I am within 10 lbs. of my ideal weight.	2	

Total Score ☐

If you do not eat meat, fish or poultry, give yourself a 2 for each meat category.

**Dark green and yellow fruits and vegetables contain beta carotene which your body can turn into vitamin A which helps protect you against certain types of cancer-causing substances.*

HOW DO YOU RATE?

0–12 A Warning Signal
Your diet is too high in fat and too low in fiber-rich foods. It would be wise to assess your eating habits to see where you could make improvements.

13–17: Not Bad! You're Partway There
You still have a way to go. Review the Dietary Guidelines below and compare them to your answers. This will help you determine where you can make a few improvements.

18–36: Good For You! You're Eating Smart
You should feel very good about yourself. You have been careful to limit your fats and eat a varied diet. Keep up the good habits and continue to look for ways to improve.

Source: *American Cancer Society,* Rev. 1989, pp. 2–5.

CHAPTER 2

The Balancing Act

THROUGH THE 1700s an illness occurred with devastating frequency among British sailors living on salt pork and hardtack during long sea voyages. Bleeding gums and dry skin first appeared, followed by sores that didn't heal but became oozing ulcers, teeth loosened and fell out, joints became excruciatingly painful, and fatigue, infections, and sometimes hysteria set in. As many as two-thirds of the men on long voyages suffered from these symptoms, and one-third died. One ship's log tells of leaving England in 1739 with 961 men on board. A year later, 626 of the men were dead. Across the ocean in the southern United States, thousands of people filled the mental institutions of the early 1900s. They suffered from a peculiar condition with no known cure—black, burnt-looking skin, severe diarrhea, dementia, and delerium. As recently as the 1950s, children growing up in poor, inner-city neighborhoods with dark tenement housing and alleyways suffered bone deformities of the legs and chest.

Today, none of these conditions is likely to occur in the United States or other industrialized countries because we now know that each was caused by the nutrient deficiencies of an inadequate diet. Sailors at sea with no fresh fruits or vegetables were suffering from scurvy, a disease caused by a vitamin C deficiency. Poor people in the south lived on greens, fatback, and cornbread, foods that lack the B vitamin niacin, and they developed the vitamin deficiency disease, pellagra. The bone deformities of rickets, caused by a deficiency of vitamin D, are seldom seen in children now because we know that sunlight, which allows skin to manufacture vitamin D, or a food source of vitamin D is necessary for healthy bones. Milk is now **fortified** with vitamin D for this reason.

Fortified: The addition of nutrients to foods in amounts greater than those naturally present in the food. Breakfast cereals and milk are foods that are most often fortified.

Although such acute, life-threatening deficiencies are now rarely seen in industrialized countries, national nutrition surveys indicate many Americans consume less than optimal quantities of certain nutrients. The Nationwide Food Consumption Survey conducted in 1977–1978 examined the nutrient intakes of approximately 40,000 Americans and found that one-third of those surveyed had low intakes of calcium, iron, magnesium, and vitamin B_6 (1). Calcium intake was especially apt to be low among women, children, and the poor. Low intakes of vitamin A and vitamin C were found in 25 percent of the individuals. Men and women between the ages of 19 and 50 took in, on average, only 56 percent of the recommended amount of zinc. The Ten-State Nutrition Survey found seriously low blood levels of **riboflavin** (a B vitamin), iron, and vitamin A among low-income people (2). Yet another large survey, the Health and Nutrition Examination Survey, found significant shortages of calcium and iron, particularly among children and women (3). These surveys and others have found undesirably low nutrient intakes to be most common among certain population groups, particularly children, women, teenagers, blacks, hispanics, and the poor.

NUTRITION BY THE NUMBERS: RECOMMENDED DIETARY ALLOWANCES

In the United States, recommended intakes of the majority of vitamins and minerals, protein, and energy are determined by the National Research Council of the National Academy of Sciences and published by the government as the **Recommended Dietary Allowances (RDAs)** (4). A vast amount of nutrition research is reviewed by this group of scientists before recommended nutrient intakes are developed. The recommendations are reviewed every few years and appropriate changes made as new information comes to light (the most recent RDAs were published in 1989). RDAs for some major nutrients are shown in table 2.1. The RDAs are not minimal amounts required to prevent deficiency diseases, but amounts considered to be "adequate to meet the known nutrient needs of practically all healthy persons." They are intended to be generous yardsticks for determining if the diets of groups of people are adequate. They are not meant to be used as rigid guidelines for individuals. Because a generous safety margin is included in setting RDAs, many individuals may meet their needs for a given nutrient by consuming only two-thirds of the RDA. RDAs are set for different age groups and

Did You Know That

The average American now drinks 62 *fewer* quarts of whole milk a year than in 1955, and 38 quarts *more* of non- or low-fat milk. This translates into a net decrease of 24 quarts of milk per person per year—and a likely calcium shortfall of about 80 milligrams a day (roughly 10 percent of the Recommended Daily Allowance).

Riboflavin: Also referred to as vitamin B_2, it is one of the B complex vitamins important in the metabolism of energy nutrients.

Recommended Dietary Allowances (RDAs): The amount of vitamins, minerals, protein, and energy that is necessary for humans to ingest daily to maintain health and energy.

Table 2.1 RDAs for Adult Men and Women

					Fat-Soluble Vitamins				Water-Soluble Vitamins		
Category	Age	Weight (lb)	Height (in)	Pro-tein (g)	Vitamin A (mcg RE)[a]	Vitamin D (mcg)	Vitamin E (mg)[b]	Vitamin K (mcg)	Vitamin C (mg)	Thia-min (mg)	Ribo-flavin (mg)
Males	15–18	145	69	59	1,000	10	10	65	60	1.5	1.8
	19–24	160	70	58	1,000	10	10	70	60	1.5	1.7
	25–50	174	70	63	1,000	5	10	80	60	1.5	1.7
	51+	170	68	63	1,000	5	10	80	60	1.2	1.4
Females	15–18	120	64	44	800	10	8	55	60	1.1	1.3
	19–24	128	65	46	800	10	8	60	60	1.1	1.3
	25–50	138	64	50	800	5	8	65	60	1.1	1.3
	51+	143	63	50	800	5	8	65	60	1.0	1.2

[a] mcg - microgram = 1/1,000,000th gram; RE - retinol equivalent = 1 mcg retinol or 6 mcg beta-carotene

[b] mg - milligram = 1/1,000th gram

Source: Food and Nutrition Board, National Academy of Sciences—National Research Council Recommended Dietary Allowances, Revised 1989.

Recommended Dietary Allowances (RDAs) are established by the National Research Council of the National Academy of Sciences and published by the government. The RDA for any given nutrient represents the amount considered "adequate to meet the known nutrient needs of practically all healthy persons."

sexes, as well as for pregnant and lactating women. You may have noticed that nutrition labels on food packages indicate the percent of the U.S. RDA of various nutrients the food provides. This variation of the RDAs is discussed in chapter 6.

FOOD GROUP GUIDES

Legumes: Dried beans and peas such as pinto, kidney, black, and navy beans. Legumes are rich in B vitamins, protein, and complex carbohydrates.

But how can we tell if our diet is adequate in nutrients without resorting to charts and numbers and time-consuming computations? Part of the solution to obtaining a diet that promotes optimal health lies in applying the principle of variety mentioned earlier. When many different types of foods are consumed, a broad range of the nutrients the body needs is more likely to be taken in each day. A person who regularly eats breads, grains, **legumes**, fruits, vegetables, meat, fish, poultry, and milk products will have better nutrient stores in his or her body and be better able to

Table 2.1 RDAs for Adult Men and Women (cont.)

Cate-gory	Age	Water-Soluble Vitamins				Minerals						
		Niacin (mg)	Vita-min B$_6$ (mg)	Folate (mcg)	Vita-min B$_{12}$ (mcg)	Cal-cium (mg)	Phos-phorus (mg)	Mag-nes-ium (mg)	Iron (mg)	Zinc (mg)	Iodine (mcg)	Sele-nium (mcg)
Males	15–18	20	2.0	200	2.0	1,200	1,200	400	12	15	150	50
	19–24	19	2.0	200	2.0	1,200	1,200	350	10	15	150	70
	25–50	19	2.0	200	2.0	800	800	350	10	15	150	70
	51 +	15	2.0	200	2.0	800	800	350	10	15	150	70
Females	15–18	15	1.5	180	2.0	1,200	1,200	300	15	12	150	50
	19–24	15	1.6	180	2.0	1,200	1,200	280	15	12	150	55
	25–50	15	1.6	180	2.0	800	800	280	15	12	150	55
	51 +	13	1.6	180	2.0	800	800	280	10	12	150	55

resist illness and disease than someone who eats mostly meat and bread, for example.

Different types of eating plans and guidelines have been in use around the world to encourage variety in food choices. In the United States a guideline based on four food groups has been in use for many years, published by the U.S. Department of Agriculture (USDA) in 1956. Other countries categorize foods into a different number of groups, but the purpose is the same—to encourage a balanced selection of a variety of foods each day.

The USDA's Daily Food Guide is shown in table 2.3, page 28. The rationale for dividing foods into the four groups is that each group provides an array of nutrients different from the others. By making a variety of choices within each group and consuming the recommended servings, an individual can be fairly certain he or she will not suffer from a severe nutrient deficiency.

For example, the fruit and vegetable group provides many vitamins and minerals, but in particular provides vitamins C and A. The bread and cereal group includes many types of grain products—breads and rolls, noodles and pasta, tortillas, cereals, rice, barley, bulgar (cracked wheat), and other cooked grains. These foods provide B vitamins, carbohydrates, and small but valuable amounts of iron and protein. The guidelines specify **enriched** or whole grain choices. The milk group, which includes cheese, yogurt and other milk products, provides calcium,

Did You Know That . . .

According to the U.S. Department of Agriculture, people over the age of 55 tend to favor more healthful snacks (fruits, cheese, and rice cakes, for example), than do younger adults.

Enriched: The addition of nutrients to foods that have lost nutrients during the process of refining. Enriched flour contains additions of niacin, riboflavin, thiamin, and iron in amounts similar to those originally present in the whole grain.

Table 2.2 Variety Counts!

Meal	A Diet With Poor Variety	A Diet With Good Variety
Break-fast	chocolate donut coffee	oatmeal with low-fat milk banana whole wheat toast with jam and butter or margarine coffee
Lunch	roast beef sandwich on white bread soft drink Oreo cookies	bean and cheese burrito rice green salad with dressing orange juice chocolate chip cookie
Snack	potato chips soft drink	strawberry yogurt
Dinner	hamburger french fries chocolate shake apple pie	baked chicken baked potato broccoli whole wheat roll with butter or margarine melon slice low-fat milk

Variety is an important element in a healthy diet. Consuming many different types of food increases a person's chance of taking in the broad range of nutrients needed by the body.

riboflavin (a B vitamin), protein, vitamin A, and in some cases vitamin D. The protein group includes meats, poultry, fish, eggs, and legumes (dried beans and peas). These foods provide protein, iron, several B vitamins, zinc, and other minerals.

For adults, the guidelines specify 4 servings daily from the bread and cereal group, 4 servings of fruits and vegetables (including selections rich in vitamin C and vitamin A), 2 servings from the protein group, and 2 from the milk group.

In a world of fast-food hamburgers, delicatessen take-out, and super supplements, guidelines based on food groups might seem an irrelevant tool. However, the Daily Food Guide does provide a good starting point for meeting important nutritional needs

---

FIGURE 2.1
How Does Your Diet Rate for Variety?

Check the box that best describes your eating habits.

How Often Do You Eat:	Seldom or Never	1 or 2 Times a Week	3 to 4 Times a Week	Almost Daily
1. At least six servings of bread, cereals, rice, crackers, pasta or other foods made from grains (a serving is one slice of bread or a half cup of cereal, rice, etc.) per day?	☐	☐	☐	☐
2. Foods made from whole grains?	☐	☐	☐	☐
3. Three different kinds of vegetables per day?	☐	☐	☐	☐
4. Cooked dry beans or peas?	☐	☐	☐	☐
5. A dark-green leafy vegetable, such as spinach or broccoli?	☐	☐	☐	☐
6. Two kinds of fruit or fruit juice per day?	☐	☐	☐	☐
7. Two servings (three if teenager, pregnant, or breastfeeding) of milk, cheese, or yogurt per day?	☐	☐	☐	☐
8. Two servings of lean meat, poultry, fish, or alternates, such as eggs, dry beans, or nuts per day?	☐	☐	☐	☐

The best answers are ALMOST DAILY for 1, 2, 3, 6, 7 and 8
3 TO 4 TIMES A WEEK for 4 and 5.

Source: Adapted from USDA *Home and Garden Bulletin* No. 232–1 (Washington, DC: Government Printing Office, April 1986).

---

daily. Keep in mind, however, that it has shortcomings as a total dietary guidance system, and you will need to apply some additional dietary wisdom. Nutritionists cite the following problems (5, 6, 7):

1. Too little iron is provided to meet the iron needs of premenopausal females and teenage boys. They need additional servings of lean meats, grains, legumes, or dark green leafy vegetables.

2. The guide's complex carbohydrate content is too low to meet the current recommendations for an increased complex carbohydrate intake. Additional servings of breads and cereals, fruits and vegetables, or legumes are needed.

(continued on p. 29)

Table 2.3 USDA Daily Food Guide

Food Group	No. of Servings a Day	Size of Serving	Notes
Vegetable and fruit group	4	½ c or a typical portion, such as 1 orange, 1 potato, etc.	Include one good source of vitamin C a day. Include deep-yellow or dark-green vegetables frequently for vitamin A. Include unpeeled fruits and vegetables for dietary fiber.
Bread and cereal group	4	1 slice bread; ½ to ¾ c cooked cereal, rice, macaroni, noodles; 1 oz ready-to-eat cereal	Include *some* whole-grain bread or cereals. Others should be enriched or fortified products.
Milk and cheese group	Children under 9: 2–3 servings Children 9–12: 3 servings Teens: 4 servings Adults: 2 servings Pregnant women: 3 servings Nursing mothers: 4 servings	8 oz milk or yogurt 1 oz cheddar or Swiss cheese = ¾ c milk ½ c ice cream = ⅓ c milk ½ c cottage cheese = ¼ c milk	Portions noted give about the same amount of calcium, but varying amounts of calories.
Meat, poultry, fish, and bean group	2	2–3 oz lean cooked meat, poultry, fish 1 egg = 1 oz meat ½ to ¾ c cooked dry beans = 1 oz meat 2 tbsp peanut butter = 1 oz meat ¼ to ½ c nuts, sesame, or sunflower seeds = 1 oz meat	Try to vary choices among these foods as each has distinct nutritional advantages. Cholesterol and vitamin B_{12} occur only in foods of animal origin, and not in plant foods.
Fats, sweets, and alcohol group	No specific recommendation. Choose foods in first four groups, then add additional foods from those groups or choose some foods from this group to reach calorie level needed	—	This group includes butter, margarine, mayonnaise, and other salad dressings; candy, sugar, jams, jellies, sweets of all kinds; soft drinks, alcoholic beverages, and unenriched, refined bakery products. These foods tend to be low in nutrients relative to their calorie contribution.

Source: *Food,* Home and Garden Bulletin No. 228, Washington, D.C.: USDA, 1979.

The United States Department of Agriculture's Daily Food Guide is a general set of dietary guidelines that was first published in 1956. It divides food into several different groups to encourage variety and thus a balanced diet.

3. The guide does not differentiate between high- and low-fat choices, high- and low-sodium choices, and high- and low-sugar choices.

4. The plan provides approximately 1200 calories, below most people's energy needs. The additional calories needed can come from more servings from the food groups or from supplemental foods (oil, butter, margarine, jam, jelly, sugar and honey, snack chips, doughnuts, desserts, soft drinks, and alcoholic beverages). However, since no guidelines are provided for the use of these supplemental foods, considerable room is left for choices that may result in a diet too high in fat, sodium, or sugar.

In one study of the plan's nutritional adequacy, an analysis of 20 menus considered good examples of the Daily Food Guide showed that less than 60 percent of the RDA was provided for vitamin E, vitamin B$_6$, magnesium, zinc, and iron (5). According to the researchers, these deficiencies can be corrected by adding daily 2 servings of legumes, a serving of a dark green leafy vegetable, 1 teaspoon of oil, and by including only whole grain breads and cereals rather than enriched.

Using the plan can be confusing for people as well. Many foods don't seem to fit easily into any one food group. The groups include foods in their minimally processed states. What about highly **processed foods**? A baked potato is a vegetable serving but what about a bag of potato chips? Is a cup of frozen yogurt a serving from the milk group? Does a doughnut qualify as a bread serving? Is a hot dog as nutritious a selection from the protein group as chicken? The answer is no to all of these and illustrates the dilemma people face in using the guidelines in our current marketplace. To remedy some of these problems, an updated version of the Daily Food Guide has been developed that provides guidelines for selecting foods that are low in fat, **cholesterol**, sodium, and sugar (6) (see table 2.4).

Using the Daily Food Guide can help you avoid underconsumption of most nutrients and, in spite of shortcomings, is a good way to determine if your diet meets the majority of vitamin, mineral, and protein needs. However, substantial concern has developed during recent years about the tendency of many Americans to consume too much of certain dietary constituents (particularly fat, sodium, protein, and sugar) and too little of other constituents (particularly complex carbohydrates and fiber).

(continued on p. 32)

Did You Know That . . .

A single 6-ounce potato contains about 40 percent of your recommended daily intake of vitamin C. It's also high in fiber, niacin, and potassium. Best of all, it has just 180 calories—if you don't add butter or sour cream.

Eating 8 ounces of potato chips, on the other hand, is like adding 12 to 20 teaspoons of vegetable oil and a teaspoon of salt to an 8-ounce potato. This is as much fat and sodium as most people should eat in an entire day.

Processed food: A food that has been treated by canning, freezing, fortification, enrichment, refining, or a change in texture.

Cholesterol: A fatlike substance found in animal foods and also manufactured by the body. It is essential to nerve and brain cell function, the synthesis of sex hormones, and is a component of bile acids used to aid fat digestion. Cholesterol is also a part of atherosclerotic plaques that accumulate on artery walls.

Table 2.4 The Basic Four, Revisited

	Anytime	Sometimes	Seldom
GRAIN GROUP *(6–11 servings a day)* **9**	Whole-grain bread*, rolls*, bagels* Whole-grain crackers*[3], tortillas* Brown rice* Bulgur Whole-grain breakfast cereal* Pasta*	Muffins*[6] Waffles, pancakes*[3] Heavily-sweetened cereals[6] Granola cereals	Croissants[3] Doughnuts[1,6] Danish[6] Bread stuffing from mix[1,3]
FRUIT & VEGETABLE GROUP *(5–9 servings a day)* **7**	All fruits and vegetables (except those at right) Applesauce, unsweetened Potatoes, white or sweet	Avocado[2], guacamole[2] Dried fruit Canned fruit[6] Fruit juice Vegetables, canned with salt[3] French fries, fried in vegetable oil[2]	Coconut[1] Pickles[3] Scalloped or au gratin potatoes[1,3] French fries, fried in beef fat[1] (McDonald's, Burger King, Wendy's)
MILK GROUP *(Children: 3–4 servings a day. Adults: 2 servings a day)* **2**	1% lowfat cottage cheese[3] Dry-curd cottage cheese Skim milk 1% lowfat milk Nonfat yogurt	2% lowfat or regular cottage cheese[3] Reduced-fat or part-skim cheeses[3] 2% lowfat milk Lowfat yogurt, plain or fruit[6] Ice milk[6] Frozen nonfat or lowfat yogurt[6]	Hard cheeses (like cheddar)[1,3] Processed cheeses[1,3] Whole milk[1] Whole-milk yogurt[1] Ice cream[1,6]

Table 2.4 The Basic Four, Revisited (cont.)

		Anytime	Sometimes	Seldom
FISH, POULTRY, MEAT, EGGS, BEANS, & NUTS GROUP *(2 servings a day)* **2**	**Fish** *(5-oz., roasted)*	All finfish[5] Salmon, canned[3,5] Sardines, in fish oil[3,5] Tuna, water-pack[3] Shellfish, except shrimp	Fried fish[2] Sardines, in vegetable oil[3] Tuna, oil-pack Shrimp[4]	
	Poultry *(4-oz., roasted)*	Chicken breast (without skin) Turkey breast, drumstick, thigh Ground turkey (without skin)	Chicken breast (with skin) Chicken drumstick, thigh Fried chicken, except thigh[2] Ground turkey (with skin)	Fried chicken thigh[2] or wing[3] Chicken hot dog[3]
	Red Meats *(3-oz., trimmed and roasted)*	Pork tenderloin	Round steak, sirloin steak Lean ham[3] Pork or lamb loin chop Leg of lamb, veal sirloin Veal loin or rib chop	Chuck blade[1], rib roast[1] Extra-lean or lean ground beef[1] Pork or lamb[1] rib chop, bacon Bologna[1,3], salami[1,3], Hot dog[1,3] Any untrimmed red meat[1]
	Eggs	Egg white		Whole egg or yolk[4]
	Beans, Peas, & Nuts	Beans, peas, lentils	Tofu[2], peanut butter[2], nuts[2]	

*refined-grain versions have less fiber, vitamins, and minerals.

[1]high in saturated fat   [2]high in unsaturated fat   [3]may be high in salt or sodium   [4]high in cholesterol
[5]may be rich in omega-3 fats   [6]high in added sugar

Source: *Nutrition Action Healthletter*, June 1990.

The Basic Four you learned in third grade never looked like this! First, we've divvied up each group into "Anytime," "Sometimes," and "Seldom" categories, according to fat, cholesterol, salt, and/or sugar levels. Next we've upped the number of servings of "Grains" to between 6 and 11 (9 on average), and increased "Fruits & Vegetables" to between 5 and 9 (7 on average).

Wondering if you'll have time to do anything but eat bread and carrots all day? Relax. The servings are quite small (1 slice of bread, 1 piece of fruit, or ½ cup of rice, pasta, or vegetables, for example).

The chart works best if you compare foods within groups (whole milk vs. skim), not between groups (rice vs. hot dogs).

Did You Know That . . .

Although heart disease remains the leading cause of death in the United States, it accounted for only 45 percent of all deaths in 1987 compared with 53 percent in 1971.

Table 2.5 Vitamin Deficiencies

Nutrient	Percent of Individuals With Intakes Less Than 70 Percent RDA
Vitamin B6	51 percent
Calcium	42 percent
Magnesium	39 percent
Iron	32 percent
Vitamin A	31 percent
Vitamin C	26 percent
Thiamin	17 percent
Vitamin B12	15 percent
Riboflavin	12 percent

Source: Robert Garrison, Jr., & Elizabeth Somer, *The Nutrition Desk Reference* (New Canaan, CT: Keats Publishing Co., 1985), 117.

Is your vitamin intake adequate? According to the 1977–78 Nationwide Food Consumption Survey, significant percentages of the population were consuming less than 70 percent of the Recommended Daily Allowance of the nutrients listed in the above table.

NEW NUTRITIONAL GUIDELINES

During the 1970s and 1980s, national health agencies and scientific councils developed guidelines to address the more recently identified dietary imbalances that contribute to the leading causes of death in the United States and other developed countries—coronary heart disease, certain types of cancer, stroke, diabetes, and **atherosclerosis**.

The widely used Dietary Guidelines for Americans (published by the U. S. Department of Agriculture and the U.S. Department of Health and Human Services) recommend (8):

Atherosclerosis: A form of hardening of the arteries in which lipids and calcium plaques gradually accumulate on artery walls, causing the blood vessels to lose elasticity and the arterial openings to narrow.

1. Eat a variety of foods.

2. Maintain desirable weight.

3. Avoid too much fat, saturated fat, and cholesterol.

4. Eat foods with adequate starch and fiber.

Table 2.6 Surveys of Nutritional Deficiencies

National Survey	Problem Nutrients	
USDA Household Food Consumption Survey, 1965–66	Vitamin A Vitamin C	Calcium
Ten State Nutrition Survey, 1968–69 (lower income groups only)	Vitamin A Vitamin C Riboflavin	Calcium Iron
First Health and Nutrition Examination Survey (HANES I), 1971–72	Vitamin A Vitamin C	Calcium Iron
USDA Nationwide Food Consumption Survey (NFCS), 1977–78	Vitamin B6 Vitamin A Vitamin C	Calcium Iron Magnesium
National Health and Nutrition Examination Survey (N-Hanes II), 1977–78	Vitamin C Thiamin Riboflavin	Iron

Source: Robert Garrison, Jr., & Elizabeth Somer, *The Nutrition Desk Reference* (New Canaan, CT: Keats Publishing Co., 1985), 117.

Major nutrition surveys conducted in the 1960s and 1970s disclosed significant micronutrient shortages among various population segments. Women, the elderly, adolescents, low-income groups, ethnic minorities, and infants and children were the groups most commonly affected.

5. Avoid too much sugar.

6. Avoid too much sodium.

7. If you drink alcoholic beverages, do so in moderation.

Recently, the National Research Council of the National Academy of Sciences issued dietary guidelines aimed at reducing risk for chronic disease (9). They are similar in many respects to the Dietary Guidelines for Americans, but more specific. Risk of developing coronary heart disease can be reduced by 20 percent if we follow these guidelines, the council states, and the risk of developing several other diseases can also be substantially reduced. The major recommendations and their rationale as outlined in the report include:

Did You Know That . . .

Although the average American has cut his or her consumption of sucrose (table sugar) to about 60 pounds a year, total per capita consumption of all types of caloric sweeteners—including corn syrup and other forms of sugar, especially those commonly used in highly processed foods, is now up to about 150 pounds per year.

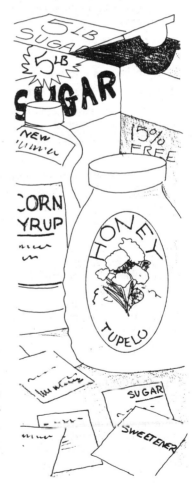

FIGURE 2.2
How Do You Score on Fat?

Do the foods you eat provide more fat than is good for you? Answer the questions below, then see how your diet stacks up.

How Often Do You Eat:	Seldom or Never	1 or 2 Times a Week	3 to 5 Times a Week	Almost Daily
1. Fried, deep-fat fried, or breaded foods?	☐	☐	☐	☐
2. Fatty meats such as bacon, sausage, luncheon meats, and heavily marbled steaks and roasts?	☐	☐	☐	☐
3. Whole milk, high-fat cheeses, and ice cream?	☐	☐	☐	☐
4. High-fat desserts such as pies, pastries, and rich cakes?	☐	☐	☐	☐
5. Rich sauces and gravies?	☐	☐	☐	☐
6. Oily salad dressings or mayonnaise?	☐	☐	☐	☐
7. Whipped cream, table cream, sour cream, and cream cheese?	☐	☐	☐	☐
8. Butter or margarine on vegetables, dinner rolls, and toast?	☐	☐	☐	☐

Take a look at your answers. Several responses in the last two columns means you may have a high fat intake. Is it time to cut back on foods high in fat?

Source: USDA *Home and Garden Bulletin* No. 232–3

Saturated fat: A type of triglyceride rich in saturated fatty acids such as stearic acid that contain no points of unsaturation in their chemical structure. Animal foods, palm oil, and coconut oil are rich in saturated fats.

Unsaturated fat: A type of triglyceride, rich in fatty acids such as oleic acid, that contains either one point of unsaturation in its chemical structure (monounsaturated) or a few points of unsaturation (polyunsaturated).

1. Reduce intake of all fats to no more than 30 percent of calories (Americans currently consume 37 percent or more of calories as fat). **Saturated fat** should provide no more than 10 percent of calories, and cholesterol should not exceed 300 milligrams daily. To achieve this, the council suggests we substitute additional complex carbohydrates and **unsaturated fats** for saturated fats. Emphasize fish, poultry without the skin, lean meats, low-fat or nonfat dairy products, and reduce fried foods, oils, fats, and fatty foods.

Rationale: Diets high in saturated fat raise blood cholesterol levels. Lowering fat consumption can reduce the risk of both heart disease and cancer.

2. Increase carbohydrate consumption to at least 55 percent of daily calories (current carbohydrate consumption is about 45

(continued on p. 36)

New Versions of Old Favorites for Heart-Healthy Diets

Supermarket shelves are overflowing with items boasting no cholesterol, and foods labeled "light." As more consumers tune in to diet and health, manufacturers will continue to turn out foods tailored to these concerns.

But buyers must beware, these claims may tell only half of the food's true nutritional story. Foods low in cholesterol, for example, may be loaded with cholesterol-raising saturated fats. Foods like peanut butter, that never had cholesterol, are labeled "no cholesterol" as if it were a breakthrough in food technology. However, many companies *are* altering their standard products, or creating tasty new foods specifically designed to meet heart-healthy guidelines. Here's a round-up of several of these new products.

EggZact, from Heart Smart Foods, is an all-natural, cholesterol-free powdered egg replacement containing 100% egg white solids and no artificial colorings or preservatives. Because it is a powder, it is shelf stable. When reconstituted with water, *EggZact* works best in baking as opposed to being used as a substitute for scrambled eggs. It is available in health food stores, or can be ordered by mail (6-ounce container, equivalent to 5 dozen eggs, $7 including postage) from Heart Smart Foods, P.O. Box 491, Needham Heights, MA 02194.

Foulds, Inc. of Libertyville, Illinois makes an egg noodle alternative called *No Yolks,* which contains no cholesterol. Regular egg noodles have 51 milligrams of cholesterol per 2-ounce serving. Though the product is currently being distributed regionally, a company spokesperson says it may be nationwide by the summer of 1990.

Cheese is a major nutritional offender, high in both cholesterol and saturated fats. Cheese lovers will welcome the variety of low-fat cheese products from First World Cheeses, producers of Alpine Lace brand reduced-fat cheeses. Tailored to the individual who wants to cut back on fat without sacrificing flavor, the newest cheese varieties are *Colbi-Lo, Monti-Jack-Lo* and *Provo-Lo.*

Compared with their whole milk equivalents, these part-skim products are lower in cholesterol and sodium, and have 5 grams of fat per ounce compared to 8 to 9 grams of fat in regular cheeses. However, not all Alpine Lace cheeses are significantly lower in fat than regular versions. *Alpine Swiss-Lo,* for example, has only 1 gram less fat than regular Swiss. So check labels to be sure that it's truly a lower-fat cheese.

The Galaxy Cheese Company, makers of Formagg brand cheese substitute, offers an array of no-cholesterol lactose-free, low-fat cheese products. Formagg is 40% lower in calories and 80% lower in saturated fats than whole milk cheeses, and is made with casein (dried skim milk protein) mixed with soybean oil. (The company says it will soon be switching to canola oil.) Jalapeno, Provolone, and Salad Topper are some of the more unusual Formagg cheese products available.

Following a heart attack, ConAgra CEO Mike Harper inspired his company to create *Healthy Choice Dinners,* a line of ten frozen microwaveable prepared meals low in fat, sodium and cholesterol. The total fat, saturated fat and cholesterol of these dinners fall within National Cholesterol Education Program recommendations, and sodium complies with 1980 National Academy of Sciences guidelines. Four new dinners are expected to be marketed soon.

Stouffer's Company has introduced *Right Course,* a line of 11 entrees similar to *Healthy Choice Dinners* in that they are all low in fat, sodium and cholesterol. The choices in this new Stouffer's line range from Fiesta Beef in Corn Pasta to Chicken in Peanut Sauce Linguini and Vegetables.

Trailblazing the snack-cake industry is Continental Baking Company's *Hostess Lights.* These no-cholesterol, iced chocolate cupcakes are designed for health-conscious eaters who occasionally enjoy a sweet snack. The new recipe was formulated substituting vegetable oil for tropical oils and animal fats, and using egg whites instead of whole eggs. There are three flavors:

plain, raspberry-filled and vanilla-pudding filled. The cakes contain 110–140 calories each. They are cholesterol-free (the originals had only 6 milligrams each) and provide only 7 to 13 percent calories from fat.

As more people cut back on saturated fat and strive to keep their cholesterol intake below the 300 milligrams daily the American Heart Association recommends, more food producers will jump on the low-fat, low-cholesterol bandwagon. Meanwhile, it's up to the consumer to scrutinize package labels and keep an eye out for new low-fat products to make healthful eating more liveable.

—*Cari Nierenberg, M.S., R.D.*

Source: Environmental Nutrition, Vol. 12, No. 12, December 1989.

Did You Know That . . .

Only 29 percent of Americans in a 1983 survey said they knew that a high-fat diet increases the risk of heart disease. By 1988, this percentage had increased to 55 percent.

percent of calories, and much of this is from sugars rather than complex carbohydrates). Eat 6 or more servings a day of starches such as rice, potatoes, pasta, whole grain breads and cereals, and legumes. Eat 5 or more servings a day of vegetables (emphasize green and yellow ones) and fruits (emphasize citrus).

Rationale: Complex carbohydrates are low in fat and calories, high in fiber and nutrients, and are the ideal replacement for fatty foods. Fruits and vegetables also contain compounds that reduce the risk for certain cancers and contain the mineral potassium, which can reduce the risk for hypertension and stroke.

3. Consume protein in moderation, eating no more than twice the amount needed. A 120-pound woman needs approximately 45 grams of protein daily, a 180-pound man approximately 65 grams.

Rationale: Protein foods tend to be high in fat and thus contribute to risk for cardiovascular disease and certain cancers. Too much protein is a factor in loss of calcium from the body and thus contributes to poor bone health.

4. Balance food intake and physical activity to maintain appropriate body weight. All healthy people should maintain a moderate level of physical activity.

Rationale: Excessive body weight contributes to the risk for diabetes, hypertension, heart disease, gallbladder disease, osteoarthritis, and endometrial cancer.

5. Alcohol consumption is not recommended. For those who do drink, limit consumption to 2 ounces of pure alcohol a day, the amount in 2 cans of beer, 2 small glasses of wine, or 2 average cocktails. Pregnant women should avoid alcohol altogether.

Rationale: Excessive alcohol intake increases the risk for heart disease, high blood pressure, chronic liver disease, some cancers, neurological diseases, and nutritional deficiencies. In addition, consumption of even small amounts of alcohol can lead to dependence.

(continued on p. 40)

Alcohol Poses Many Health Risks, Few Benefits

In the 1920's alcohol was considered evil and illegal. Today's concerns about alcohol focus on its health effects. While some studies show it may help prevent heart disease, others have linked it to breast cancer, high blood pressure and birth defects. Are there medical reasons to imbibe or to avoid alcohol completely?

Alcohol and Blood Pressure. Excessive alcohol intake may be the most common cause of secondary hypertension (high blood pressure for which the cause is known). U.S. population studies show 3 to 10 percent of high blood pressure in men is due to alcohol; in women, the percentage is lower. One obvious reason for the lower incidence of alcohol-induced hypertension in women is that fewer women drink. A more important reason may be that women react differently to alcohol.

Whereas the relationship between alcohol intake and blood pressure in men is linear—the more alcohol consumed, the higher the blood pressure—the relationship in women is U-shaped. That is, women who drink moderately (up to 20 grams of alcohol a day—the equivalent of about 8 ounces of wine) tend to have lower blood pressures than abstainers (1), while those who drink more have more hypertension.

In general, hypertension is 1.6 to 2.4 times more prevalent in heavy drinkers than in non-drinkers (1). But heavy drinking is defined in various ways in various studies, making study comparisons difficult. According to Michael J. Klag, M.D., M.P.H., Assistant Professor in the Department of Epidemiology at the Johns Hopkins Medical Institutions, at a level above three drinks a day, most people will experience a rise in blood pressure—4 to 6 points systolically (the top number in a blood pressure reading) and 2 to 3 points diastolically (the bottom number). Although these numbers may seem small, Dr Klag stresses they are averages. "Some people will see less of an effect; others will experience higher blood pressures."

Alcohol and Heart Disease. Not all the news about alcohol is bad. Some studies suggest moderate drinking reduces people's risk of incurring the nation's #1 killer, heart disease. While previous studies have focused almost exclusively on men, a recent study has confirmed that alcohol reduces womens' risk, too. The Nurse's Health Study of 87,000 women, found that those drinking three to nine drinks a week had a 40 percent lower risk of heart disease compared to non-drinkers. (2) The study also found moderate drinkers to have a 30 percent lower risk of ischemic strokes (strokes due to blockage of blood vessels in the brain).

Researchers believe that alcohol may exert its protective effect by increasing levels of high density lipoproteins in the blood—the "good" cholesterol that helps protect against heart disease. It may also decrease slightly the blood's tendency to clot, thereby producing a protective effect against strokes caused by blood clots.

According to the Nurse's Health Study, however, drinking increases a woman's risk of a less common form of stroke. Hemorrhagic stroke (stroke from bleeding) was found to be two to three times more common in women who drank moderately.

In men, alcohol's effect on stroke risk is unclear, primarily because it hasn't been studied extensively. One study of men, the Honolulu Heart Program, showed that male drinkers, like women, experienced a two or three times greater risk of hemorrhagic stroke, but found no evidence of alcohol protecting them against ischemic stroke. (3)

Alcohol and Breast Cancer. One of the most highly publicized detrimental effects of alcohol also came from the Nurse's Health Study. It found that drinkers experienced a 30 percent increase in the risk for breast cancer. But according to Clark Heath, Vice President of Epidemiology and Statistics at the American Cancer Society, this is just one in a series of studies that disagree about alcohol's impact on breast cancer. "The data aren't so strong that you should worry if you have one drink a day," says Mr. Clark.

Meir Stampfer, M.D. Associate Physician at the Brigham and Women's Hospital in Boston and one of the principal investigators in the Nurse's Health Study, adds further perspective to the conflict: "Heart disease kills far more women than breast cancer. On the other hand, we don't know how to prevent breast cancer, while there are lots of ways to prevent heart disease."

Fetal Alcohol Syndrome. When it comes to drinking during pregnancy, experts generally agree there's no such thing as a safe amount of alcohol for women. Fetal alcohol syndrome (FAS) is among the three leading known causes of birth defects resulting in mental retardation. And it is the only preventable one among them.

Full blown fetal alcohol syndrome, with its accompanying physical and mental abnormalities, has been reported in infants of women who consumed as few as two drinks a day, according to Agnes Huber, Ph.D., R.D. immediate past president of the Nutrition and Dietetics Division of the American Association of Mental Retardation.

Alcohol negatively affects the developing fetus in two ways: It collapses blood vessels, depriving the fetus of oxygen and glucose, and it dries out cells, destroying neurons and damaging the developing brain.

What about the woman who drinks in the early weeks of pregancy, before she is aware she's expecting? The best advice, according to Dr. Huber, is to stop drinking as soon as she knows she is pregnant. Not every fetus whose mother drinks will have FAS. In fact, most infants of women who drink will not develop FAS. But because experts can't identify those who will, they recommend that women not drink at all during pregnancy.

Although alcohol has long been and is still promoted as an aid to breastfeeding, Dr. Huber advises against it. Alcohol is secreted in the breast milk and brain cells continue to be formed until a child is about two years of age.

To Drink or Not. Conflicting studies are the rule rather than the exception in alcohol research, primarily because of differences in the definition of what constitutes a drink, the number of drinks that make a person a "heavy drinker" and how accurate a person's recall is of his previous drinking.

Despite the conflicting findings, most experts agree that any possible health benefits from alcohol are small, and some feel its negative effects far outweigh any positive ones. The general consensus, then is that drinking's health benefits are neither cause to start drinking, nor should they be used as an excuse to continue doing so.

—*Marsha Hudnall, M.S., R.D.*

(1) *Postgraduate Medicine,* pp. 273–274, June, 1984.
(2) *The New England Journal of Medicine,* pp. 273–276, August 4, 1988.
(3) *Journal of the American Medical Association,* pp. 2311–2314, May 2, 1986.

What Is a Drink?

Although definitions vary, researchers frequently define a single drink as one that contains 13 grams of alcohol. That translates into:

Drink	Amount of Ounces
Lite beer	14
Regular beer	12
Wine	5
Bloody Mary	4.6
Coffee liqueur	1.7
Creme de Menthe	1.3
80 proof rum, vodka or bourbon	1.3

Source: *Environmental Nutrition,* Vol. 12, No. 7, July 1989.

Table 2.7 Top 20 Cancer-Fighting Foods

	Serv-ing Size	Vita-min A* (IU)	Vita-min C (mg)	Cal-cium (mg)	Fiber (g)	Sele-nium (mcg)
Apricots, fresh	3	2,770	11	15	2	n/a**
Broccoli, fresh	1/2 cup	1,100	49	89	3	0
Brussels sprouts	1/2 cup	560	48	28	3	5
Cabbage	1/2 cup	70	18	25	2	0
Cantaloupe, 5" diameter	1/2	8,610	113	29	3	0
Carrots	1/2 cup	19,150	2	24	3	1
Chicken, skinless	3 oz	50	0	0	0	10
Collards, frozen	1/2 cup	5,080	22	178	2	n/a
Flounder	3.5 oz	100	0	29	0	85
Haddock	3.5 oz	150	0	55	0	34
Milk, skim	8 oz	1,490	2	302	0	12
Orange juice, fresh	8 oz	500	124	27	1	1
Peppers, sweet, red, raw	1	4,220	141	4	1	1
Pumpkin, canned	1/2 cup	27,020	5	32	2	n/a
Roll, whole-wheat	1	10	0	25	4	23
Shrimp	3.5 oz	180	0	320	0	54
Squash, butter-nut, fresh, cooked	1/2 cup	7,170	15	42	2	1
Sweet po-tatoes, baked	4 oz	24,880	28	32	3	1
Tomatoes	1	1,390	22	9	2	1
Tuna, canned in water	3 oz	320	0	17	0	73

*The Vitamin A in fruits and vegetables comes primarily from beta-carotene

**n/a = Not Available

Sources: Charts: ESHA Database; U.S. Department of Agriculture Handbooks 8–5, 8–10, 8–13, 456; Pennington and Church's *Food Values of Portions Commonly Used*, 14th Ed.; and product labels. From article by D. Webb, "Cut Your Cancer Risk by More Than 50%," *Redbook* (April 1989), pp. 96–99, 149.

Chock Full of Fiber

Eat more of the following and you may reduce your risk of colon cancer.

	Fiber (g)
Pinto beans, dried, cooked, 1/2 cup	10
Wheat bran, 1/2 cup	8
Raisins, 1/2 cup	6
Cereal, bran, 1 cup	4–24
Peas, canned, 1/2 cup	5
Potato, with skin, 1 small	4
Raspberries, 1/2 cup	4
Apple, peeled, 1 me-dium	4
Corn, canned, 1/2 cup	3
Orange, fresh, Califor-nia navel, 1	3
Bran muffin, 1	3
Bread, whole-wheat, 1 slice	2

Best-Bet Dairy

Dairy products are loaded with cal-cium) the "newest" cancer-pre-ventive nutrient. The items below—all low in fat—are smart selections.

	Cal-cium (mg)
Milk, evaporated skim, canned, 8 oz	738
Yogurt, low-fat or non-fat, plain, 8 oz	450
Milk, skim, 8 oz	302
Milk, 1% milkfat, 8 oz	300
Milk, 1% milkfat, choc-olate, 8 oz	287
Buttermilk, 8 oz	285
Ice milk, 5.1% milkfat, 1 cup	204
Yogurt drink, low-fat, flavored, 8 oz	200

While we do not yet have answers to many of the questions concerning which types of food may provide some protection against the development of cancer, most experts agree that there are ways to apply what we do know. One of these ways is to increase the consumption of foods such as those shown above which are both generally nutritious and currently thought to be of some value in preventing cancer.

6. Limit daily salt intake to 6 grams or less (about a teaspoon). Limit the salt used in cooking and added to food at the table. Consume small amounts of salty, highly processed salty, and salt-pickled foods.

Rationale: Diets containing more than 6 grams of salt a day are associated with high blood pressure. Additionally, salt-pickled foods are suspected of increasing the risk for stomach cancer.

7. Maintain adequate calcium intake. Consume low-fat or nonfat milk products and dark green vegetables.

Rationale: Calcium is an essential nutrient often low in diets, particularly in the diets of women and adolescents. Low calcium intake is associated with increased risk for **osteoporosis** and bone fractures and possibly high blood pressure.

Cancer prevention guidelines issued by the Committee on Diet, Nutrition, and Cancer of the National Academy of Sciences also recommend Americans reduce fat intake to no more than 30 percent of calories (10). They recommend, in addition, that we frequently consume whole grain products (for fiber), citrus fruits (for vitamin C), carotene-rich fruits and vegetables (colored deep yellow, orange, and dark green) and cruciferous vegetables (broccoli, brussel sprouts, cabbage and cauliflower), minimize intake of salt-cured, salt-pickled and smoked foods, and avoid excessive alcohol consumption, especially in conjunction with cigarette smoking.

Use the self-assessments on pages 18–21, 27, 34 to see how your diet measures up and where you can most beneficially make changes. At first glance, it might seem that making dietary changes to meet all of these recommendations is a big task. However, small changes are often all that is needed, and improving one area of the diet tends to have a domino effect in leading to improvement of other areas. Throughout the following chapters you will find information to help you develop a diet that meets current guidelines for maintaining health and preventing chronic disease. W

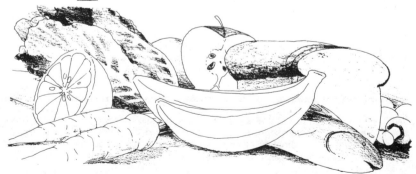

Osteoporosis: A condition of weak, porous bones resulting from loss of bone density over time.

Can Eating the 'Right' Food Cut Your Risk of Cancer?

"About one-third of all cancer deaths may be related to what we eat." "150,000 lives could be saved annually through dietary changes." "More than four of five adult Americans know that eating the wrong foods may increase their chances of developing some kinds of cancer." These are some of the bold pronouncements made during the last few years by such prestigious organizations as the American Cancer Society and the National Cancer Institute. Granted, the statements are usually tempered by qualifiers like "these estimates cannot be considered definitive" and "the evidence is incomplete." Nonetheless, the underlying message that what we eat has a direct bearing on the risk for developing cancer has come through loud and clear. And the connection has been further popularized by advertisements for a variety of products implying, for example, that certain kinds of cereals may ward off colon cancer and certain nutritional supplements will act as "protector vitamins."

Would that it were so simple: Eat a specific food. Swallow a specific pill. And prevent cancer.

An enormous amount of research is going on worldwide. And while there is gathering evidence to support the links between what you eat day-to-day and the long-term development of cancer—particularly cancer of the breast and the colon—there also is a growing body of conflicting evidence emerging that these links are not so specific. All of this, in turn, is fueling a behind-the-scenes debate within the scientific community over whether the public is being misled into believing something that may not be quite true.

A host of practical questions are being raised. Is it a good idea to decrease the amount of fat you eat to a minimum and increase the amount of fiber to keep cancer at bay, as many advocates of these measures advise? Or is that ill-founded advice? What about those so-called protector nutrients? Should you eat more of the foods that contain these substances? Are supplements in order? Although science has not yet come up with "yes" or "no" answers to these questions, an examination of what is known should help

concerned readers put the issues into perspective.

What's the evidence on breast cancer?

Breast cancer has become the leading cancer killer of women. In 1985, the latest year for which reliable figures are available, more than 40,000 women in the United States died of the disease. Against the backdrop of this distressing statistic, scientists are debating whether women can reverse the trend by cutting back on the percentage of fat in their meals.

Those who advocate a low-fat diet to reduce the incidence of breast cancer have much to back them up. In fact, of all the suggested links between diet and cancer, "the association between dietary fat and breast cancer comes closest to fulfilling the criteria" epidemiologists look for when they make inferences about what causes disease, says Leonard A. Cohen, PhD, of the American Health Foundation in Valhalla, New York.

What has been found by studying population groups is that Japanese women who eat a traditional Japanese diet—about 20 percent of its total calories come from fat—are significantly less apt to fall victim to breast cancer than women in countries such as the United States, where the diet is high in fat. Indeed, breast cancer has been estimated to be four to five times as common in the U.S. as in Japan.

Particularly telling is the evidence gathered on the granddaughters and great-granddaughters of Japanese families who migrated to Hawaii and the mainland of the United States and adopted a diet higher in fat. The breast cancer rates among these Americanized women approaches that of other women in the country. Indeed, it took only a couple of generations for the increase in breast cancer to occur. The same is true for American-born women of Polish descent. They have a higher breast cancer rate than their ancestors, who ate a lower-fat diet. Clearly, genetic determinants cannot be the sole influencers.

Adding weight to the hypothesis that a high-fat diet carries with it an increased risk of breast cancer is the fact that in Japan today, where the national cuisine is quickly becoming "western-ized" and, thus, higher in fat content, the inci-dence of breast cancer is on the rise.

Despite this evidence, there are those who cautiously point out that none of the studies linking fat to breast cancer provide absolute proof of a cause-and-effect relationship. And they are correct. Epidemiological comparisons cannot serve as a "bottom line." For while they show that women in countries with low-fat diets have a lower incidence of breast cancer than women in countries with high-fat diets, they do not rule out the possibility that other environmental influ-ences or genetic variations account for the differ-ence. Studies on laboratory animals cannot serve as a bottom line either. Even though they indicate that a reduced fat intake decreases the incidence of mammary tumors in rodents, they cannot automatically be extrapolated to humans.

As if to cast even more doubt on a connection between fat and breast cancer, skeptics also point to a recently completed Harvard study of almost 90,000 women, which revealed that those who took in 44 percent of their calories from fat were no more likely to develop breast cancer than those who consumed only 32 percent of their calories from fat.

But is 32 percent fat low enough? Not accord-ing to scientists whose research suggests that the risk of breast cancer does not decrease little by little as fat is gradually cut out of the diet but, instead, there is a cutoff point below which women are not at high risk for breast cancer and above which they are. In effect there may be what they term a "threshold" point. Not all propo-nents of the threshold effect agree on just where the cutoff point lies, but many believe it is *below* 30 percent of calories as fat. Sherwood L. Gor-bach, MD, a professor of medicine at Tufts who has conducted numerous studies on the link between diet and breast cancer, recommends a diet consisting of 20 to 25 percent fat calories. He is not convinced, however, that the threshold effect should rule women's thinking about lower-ing fat calories and believes that "to whatever

extent you can lower your fat intake, you might be lowering your breast cancer risk." And even though the conclusion reached at Harvard ques-tions such a view, he notes that that study may have its own inherent flaws, just as epidemiologi-cal observations do, and cannot be taken as final.

Also particularly disappointing to Dr. Gorbach as well as many others is the decision just made by the National Cancer Institute to cancel a massive $130 million study involving 30,000 women that was supposed to determine whether a 20 percent fat diet could reduce the incidence of breast cancer in 45- to 69-year-old women by half in 10 years. "Now," he says, "we will have no proof of preventive measures, only detection measures once the cancer has developed."

Dr. Peter Greenwald, the director of the Na-tional Cancer Institute's Division of Cancer Pre-vention and Control, does not dispute the claim that too much fat in the diet may contribute to an increased risk of breast cancer. But "after 40 years of research," he says, "we do not have a clear consensus." And for now, the NCI is staying with its original public message, which is to decrease fat intake to no more than 30 percent of total calories and to maintain desirable weight.

What is a woman who wants to protect herself from losing a breast or, worse yet, her life to make of all this? Should she follow the recommenda-tion to lower fat intake to 30 percent of total calories, which is also the advice for lowering the risk of heart disease, by reducing her intake of butter, oils, high-fat meats, dairy products, and snacks? Or should she reduce it to somewhere in the 20 percent range?

While no one can answer those questions definitively, it should be pointed out that it is certainly better for heart health, if for nothing else, to lower fat intake from 40 percent of total calories, which is what American women are accustomed to, to 30 percent. There is no harm in decreasing fat intake to 25 or even 20 percent of total calories, as the traditional Japanese diet shows. But it would be difficult for a woman used to a 40 percent fat diet to suddenly cut that percentage in half, since the changes likely to "stick" when it comes to diet are the gradual ones.

In addition to lowering the risk of heart disease, a low fat intake appears to help in decreasing the incidence of cancers of the pancreas and ovaries. And since fat contributes two or three times as many calories as protein and carbohydrates (including the simple carbohydrate sugar), reducing intake is likely to help overweight women shed excess pounds.

What's the evidence on colon cancer?

The protective effect gained from reducing fat intake is also speculated to lower the chance of falling victim to colon cancer, the second leading cause of cancer death in the United States among males and females combined. (The leading cause of death from cancer is lung cancer.) The supposition stems, in part, from research demonstrating that a high intake of fat causes greater secretion of bile acids. And while bile acids are necessary to help the body digest fats, they have also been shown to promote tumors in the colon, or large bowel, in laboratory animals. Dietary fiber appears to minimize the harmful effects of bile acids and thereby inhibit tumor development, according to some researchers. But it has not yet been determined whether an increased fiber intake works independently of decreased fat intake or whether the two must operate in tandem for an optimal anti-cancer effect. In either case, fiber is thought to help decrease risk in one or more ways: increasing the bulk of stool, which may dilute the concentration of cancer-causing agents; speeding the passage of stool through the colon and thereby lessening the time carcinogens or carcinogenic substances in waste can do damage; and binding to carcinogens that might otherwise remain free to work on producing a tumor.

Despite these theories, "the data concerning fiber and cancer are still inconsistent," says Lucien Jacobs, MD, of Los Angeles's Cedars-Sinai Medical Center. In fact, he warns, "a high level of intake of certain kinds of fiber could be deleterious." One of the hitches is that there are many different types of fiber, and not all types appear to be protective. While the insoluble fiber present in whole-wheat products has held up relatively consistently as a cancer inhibitor in research on rats, the soluble fibers found in oat bran and fruits have been shown to *stimulate* tumor production in laboratory experiments by increasing the concentration of bile acids.

To make matters even more confusing, Greenland Eskimos, who eat no fiber to speak of but whose diets are extremely high in fat, have a low rate of colon cancer. And studies on vegetarians, who normally consume relatively large quantities of fiber and suffer less than others from colon cancer, show they may be more disposed to developing stomach cancer.

All these seeming inconsistencies might lead to the conclusion that "you're damned if you do and damned if you don't." But closer examination reveals that the type of fat Greenland Eskimos eat consists largely of the omega-3 fatty acids found in fish, which may not have the same effect on the secretion of bile acids as the typical saturated and polyunsaturated fats of the American diet. As for vegetarians, the amount of fiber they eat may throw off the stomach's acid-alkaline equilibrium and thereby heighten the risk of developing cancer. Or, fiber may increase cell proliferation in certain cases, thus giving tumors greater opportunity for development. It is even possible that the epidemiological associations between fiber and stomach cancer are spurious, that is, they have no real biological basis.

That's not to say that the data on stomach cancer should be dismissed. It simply underscores the fact that while the epidemiological and laboratory findings on the relationship between fiber, fat, and various cancers are provocative, the final word is not yet in and perhaps won't be for many years. In short, it cannot be said unequivocally that fiber protects against colon cancer or paves the way for stomach cancer or, indeed, has any definite effect on cancerous tumors. Anyone who implies otherwise has gone beyond the limits of what scientific studies have proven so far.

"It's going to take a lot more research to get it straightened out," says David Kritchevsky of Philadelphia's Wistar Institute. For all we know, he adds, fiber's role in preventing colon cancer might just be to limit calorie intake. He has found that restricting calorie intake in rats reduces the incidence and size of tumors, and he suggests that perhaps fiber helps ward off colon cancer not by some elaborate mechanism but simply by contributing to over-all calorie restriction. (Theoretically, the more calorie-less fiber consumed, the less room there is for calorie-dense foods, including foods high in fat.)

Such uncertainties may not sit well with the health-conscious consumer who is eager to eat the "right" amount of fiber. One thing is clear, however. The average daily fiber intake of U.S. adults is only 11 grams, according to a national survey. What's more, half of the adults in this country consume fewer than 10 grams of fiber a day. A sampling of those typical diets has revealed that they are generally devoid of whole-grain products (a source of insoluble fiber) and contain two or fewer servings of vegetables and/or fruits (sources of soluble fiber). Clearly, the American population at large can afford to add some whole-grain breads and cereals along with vegetables, fruits, and high-fiber legumes and nuts to the diet without worrying that they will take in *too much* roughage, either soluble or insoluble. At the most, such a change will reduce the risk of such devastating illnesses as colon cancer. At the least, they will insure more regular bowel movements and increase consumption of the essential vitamins and minerals in produce and whole-grain foods.

Vitamins: Does more mean better?

In the 1970s, Norwegian men who smoked and who also had low amounts of vitamin A in their diets were shown to run a higher risk for developing lung cancer than others who did not. Similarly, observation of 250,000 people over the course of a decade in Japan uncovered what appeared to be a link between daily consumption of vegetables that are high in beta-carotene, a compound in plant foods that is converted to vitamin A in the body, and a decreased risk of cancers of the lung, colon, stomach, prostate, and cervix. Such studies abound. In one study at Johns Hopkins University, 99 people who developed lung cancer had 14 percent less beta-carotene in their blood than 200 other people who had remained free of the disease. Not only

that, their blood contained 12 percent less vitamin E.

What is it about substances like beta-carotene and vitamin E that seems to enable them to ward off different types of cancers? More to the point, if they are so beneficial, should people now ignore the recommended dietary allowances and begin taking super-large quantities of these compounds? No one knows for certain what the potentially protective properties of beta-carotene and vitamin E are, but researchers think they may be instrumental in blocking the action of certain highly reactive chemical entities in the body that can alter the normal functioning of cells and thereby set the stage for tumors to develop in various tissues.

To find out more about whether beta-carotene and vitamin E play a role in preventing cancer—and if they do, how so—scientists are conducting studies known as chemoprevention trials, in which large numbers of people are given supplemental doses of one or more substances and observed over a period of several years to see if they are less likely to succumb to cancer than others. Some 23,000 male physicians throughout the U.S., for example, are participating in a trial funded by the National Cancer Institute to determine if beta-carotene supplements will decrease the overall incidence of cancer. Other groups are being given vitamin E. In no way, however, does the Institute mean for people to misconstrue such ongoing research, the results of which will not be known until the 1990s, as a go-ahead to take megadoses of beta-carotene, vitamin E, vitamin A, or any other nutrient. NCI's Dr. Greenwald points out that the evidence on the ability of various vitamins and minerals to reduce cancer risk comes from observations of people's patterns of *food* intake. Therefore, there is no justification, research or not, for anyone to practice chemoprevention on himself.

Indeed, while large doses of beta-carotene are relatively harmless, too much vitamin A can cause permanent liver damage. And selenium, a mineral that is also thought to have some anti-cancer properties and is being tested in chemoprevention studies, can be toxic in amounts easily obtainable from pills. Even vitamin C, which is seemingly harmless at high dosages and which some people take in tablets containing 10 to 15 times the RDA of 60 milligrams, is a cause of concern for professionals because the safety of taking huge amounts of the vitamin is by no means certain. It is true that vitamin C, which like beta-carotene and vitamin E may be able to "deactivate" reactive chemical entities in the body and thereby ward off cancer, is being given in supplemental form in chemoprevention research to see if it can halt the onset or growth of tumors. But the levels of that nutrient and others administered to study participants often amount to pharmacological doses that must be monitored by physicians. They should not be thought of as innocuous, especially because even the doctors conducting the studies are not certain about what their outcomes will be.

The bottom line? Try to get a good supply of the vitamins and other substances that show promise of being able to keep cancer at bay from foods: beta-carotene from deep orange and yellow and dark green fruits and vegetables; vitamin C from almost any bin in the produce aisle; vitamin E from the vegetable oils used (sparingly) in cooking; and selenium from seafood and organ meats. Many of these have the added bonus of being high in fiber and low in fat, so by eating the varied diet that is necessary for obtaining all these nutrients, you may be keeping yourself healthy in many ways at once.

Foods to pick, changes to make

While not all the answers are in yet as far as which dietary components may protect against or contribute to the development of various kinds of cancer, most experts agree that by following a particular pattern in making food choices, health-conscious eaters will be applying the best of what has been gleaned so far about reducing the chance of developing cancer through dietary measures. If it turns out that the dietary pattern

does not decrease the chances of developing cancer as much as many scientists hope, at least it will provide the balance of nutrients that is essential to the maintenance of general health as well as assist in the fight against heart disease and obesity. The prescribed pattern:

- Eat fewer items that are high in fat, including meats with a good deal of marbeling, fried foods, cold cuts such as bologna and salami, bacon, whole milk and cream, creamed dishes, rich desserts, and meals prepared with lots of oil, butter, or margarine.
- Consume more low-fat dairy products, such as low-fat yogurt, cottage cheese, and skim milk, baked or broiled poultry without the skin, fish, and lean cuts of meat with all visible fat trimmed away.
- Select fiber-rich whole-grain breads, cereals, and pastas (the ingredients list must contain the words *whole-wheat* or *whole-grain*), all manner of fruits and vegetables, legumes, oat-based products, and, in moderation, nuts (which are relatively high in fat).
- Increase daily intake of fruits and vegetables rich in beta-carotene, like cantaloupe, apricots, sweet potatoes, spinach, and broccoli.
- Eat a variety of produce that contains appreciable amounts of vitamin C, which includes everything from citrus fruits to strawberries to dark green leafy vegetables.
- Get enough vitamin E by using small amounts of polyunsaturated oils when cooking and by eating a wide variety of vegetables.
- Make seafood a regular part of the weekly diet to insure an adequate intake of selenium. Organ meats provide selenium, too, but they also provide a lot of fat and cholesterol, so they should be eaten only occasionally.

Source: *Tufts University Diet & Nutrition Letter*, Vol. 6, No. 2, April 1988.

Game Plan For A Healthy Diet

The Nutrients • Energy Balance • Carbohydrates

OODS CONTAIN AN AMAZING array of flavor substances, pigments, fibers, hormones, chemicals for self-defense against insects and viruses, pharmacological and medicinal compounds, naturally occurring toxicants and nutrients. In the study of nutrition we look primarily at the last category, but the nonnutrient substances in food can have a profound effect on health as well. At present, the balance and interactions between all the various components in food are a vast and fascinating area only partially understood.

MEET THE PLAYERS: THE NUTRIENTS

Nutrients are substances in food that build and sustain bodily tissues and are required for bodily functions. They are divided into six major categories: water, carbohydrates, proteins, lipids (fats), vitamins, and minerals. The body is able to manufacture some nutrients, and these are termed nonessential nutrients. Those that the body cannot make at all, or cannot make in sufficient quantity to support health, are termed essential nutrients—they must be obtained from the diet.

The nutrients work in three ways: they are burned or oxidized to furnish energy (carbohydrates, proteins, and lipids); they become building materials for the maintenance and repair of cells, tissues, and organs (proteins, lipids, minerals, water); and they act as "traffic police" to help regulate cellular reactions and other bodily processes (proteins, vitamins, minerals, water).

At the present time, 13 vitamins and at least 15 minerals are considered essential nutrients for humans—they are required for life, are not manufactured by the body, and must be taken in

Nutrients: Compounds used by the body for growth, maintenance, and repair. Nutrients are essential to life and most cannot be manufactured by the body and must be taken in through food.

46

The Nutrients

- **Macronutrients:** Used for fuel, needed in large quantities—

   Carbohydrate
   Protein
   Lipid (fat)

- **Micronutrients:** Needed in small quantities—

   Vitamins
   Major minerals (more than 100 mg per day needed)
   Minor minerals and trace elements (less than 100 mg per day needed)

- **Water**

through the diet. These, and other elements currently thought to be of nutritional importance, are listed in the box on page 48.

As mentioned earlier, consuming a healthy diet doesn't require keeping track of all the milligrams and grams and calories of nutrients that are eaten, but rather incorporating a balanced intake of different foods into one's eating pattern (after all, we eat foods, not numbers!). A first step is to consume a diet that provides well-balanced proportions of the nutrients that supply energy or calories: carbohydrates, fats, and proteins.

ENERGY BALANCE: THE INS AND OUTS

The First Law of Thermodynamics, which states energy is neither created nor destroyed but only converted from one form to another, applies to the human body as much as to the rest of the universe. We take in energy in the form of food and either convert that energy into heat as we "burn" it or we store it as fat or other tissue (as any overweight person will lament!). Consuming enough foods to meet the body's need for energy is the first requirement for being well-nourished.

Energy value in foods is measured in kilocalories, although this is often shortened to just calories. A person is said to be in

What We Know About Nutrients

Recommended Dietary Allowances (RDAs) are provided for the following nutrients

Protein	B vitamins:	Minerals:
vitamin A	thiamin	calcium
vitamin D	riboflavin	phosphorus
vitamin E	niacin	magnesium
vitamin K	vitamin B6	iron
vitamin C	folate	zinc
	vitamin B12	iodine
		selenium

Estimated Safe and Adequate Daily Dietary Intakes (not enough is known about these to determine RDAs)

biotin	fluoride
pantothenic acid	chromium
copper	molybdenum
manganese	

Trace Elements in Diet Probably Needed by Humans

silicon	arsenic
tin	nickel
vanadium	

Additional Trace Elements in Diet, Functions Unknown

barium	cadmium
bromine	gold
strontium	silver
aluminum	mercury
bismuth	gallium
lead	antimony
boron	lithium

energy balance or equilibrium when the calories consumed through food are equivalent to the calories expended by the body and weight is neither gained nor lost. Children, pregnant women, and athletes building new muscle are in a state of positive energy balance—they are taking in more calories than they expend and the extra calories consumed are used to build new tissue.

Undernourished people and those actively losing weight are in negative energy balance. They are taking in fewer calories

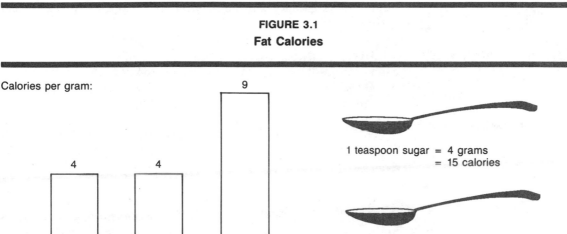

FIGURE 3.1
Fat Calories

Calories per gram:

9

4   4

Carbohydrates   Proteins   Fats

1 teaspoon sugar = 4 grams
= 15 calories

1 teaspoon fat = 4.5 grams
= 40 calories

Fat is more than twice as concentrated in calories as carbohydrate or protein. A single gram of fat contains 9 calories versus 4 calories for a gram of carbohydrate or protein.

A teaspoon of fat contains nearly three times as many calories as a teaspoon of sugar, 40 versus 15.

than they are expending, and body tissues are being broken down to supply the additional energy required.

A person's energy or calorie requirement results from three needs: energy required to fuel the body's vital functions while at rest (termed the basal metabolic rate), energy needed for physical activity, and energy needed to digest and absorb food.

The **basal metabolic rate** varies between individuals depending on several factors, including age, body weight, muscle mass, gender, and body shape. A rough formula for calculating basal metabolic expenditure is to multiply one's weight in kilograms (pounds divided by 2.2) by 24. The resulting figure is an estimate of the basal metabolic calories needed daily (1).

For inactive or moderately active people, the calories needed for basal metabolism make up as much as 70 percent or more of the total daily calorie needs. Very active people and athletes, however, may need just as many calories to meet their needs for physical activity. For example, a 140-pound woman who walks to and from campus, runs for an hour and bicycles for an hour each day may have a basal metabolic expenditure of 1536 calories but may require an additional 1300 calories to support physical activity. A second 140-pound woman with the same basal metabolic expenditure who has a desk job and is not physically active

Basal metabolic rate: The energy required to keep the body functioning at rest (to maintain breathing, heart-heat, body temperature, and other bodily functions). The metabolic rate increases in response to exertion, stress, fear, and illness. Also referred to as metabolic rate.

might require only an additional 400 calories for physical activity.

The energy requirement for digesting and absorbing food is relatively small, approximately 10 percent of the basal metabolic calories and physical activity calories added together. The combined total of basal metabolic calories, physical activity calories, and calories needed to assimilate food equals a person's total daily caloric requirement. Using the example of the active woman above, we can determine the calorie requirement as 1536 + 1300 + 284 (.10 × 1536 + 1300) for a total requirement of 3120 calories.

The RDA for calories for the average woman engaged in light to moderate activity is estimated to be 2200 calories a day and for the average man, 2900 calories (2). The actual number of calories an individual needs, of course, may be higher or lower depending primarily on body size and activity level.

Overweight

It is estimated at least 20 to 30 percent of the population in the United States is above their desirable body weight, increasing risk for cardiovascular disease, hypertension, diabetes, gallbladder disease, osteoarthritis, and certain cancers (3). At the same time, surveys indicate the average caloric intake of women is only 1560 calories, far below the estimated average need of 2200 calories (2). Considering the high incidence of overweight in the population, this indicates we are, on the whole, extraordinarily inactive!

Overweight can only occur when one has consumed more calories than the body is expending on a daily basis. The excess calories, whether from protein, carbohydrate, fat, or alcohol, are changed into a storage form of fat and placed in adipose (fat) tissue. The solution to the overweight dilemma is either to take in fewer calories or expend more calories, or both. Neither appetite suppressants, fiber pills, grapefruit pills, cellulite treatments, hormone injections, body wraps, herbal formulas, restricted carbohydrate diets, crash diets, nor diets specifying certain food combinations are successful approaches to fat loss, although some may result in temporary weight loss (often of muscle and water, not fat).

A pound of body fat contains 3500 calories. If a person consumes 250 calories fewer each day and expends 250 calories more through physical activity for a net deficit of 500 calories daily, approximately a pound of fat can be lost in a week.

Many people attempt to lose weight solely through cutting

Table 3.1 Desirable Body Weight Ranges

MEN					WOMEN				
Height Feet	Inches	Small Frame	Medium Frame	Large Frame	Height Feet	Inches	Small Frame	Medium Frame	Large Frame
5	2	128–134	1131–141	138–150	4	10	102–111	109–121	118–131
5	3	130–136	133–143	140–153	4	11	103–113	111–123	120–134
5	4	132–138	135–145	142–156	5	0	104–115	113–126	122–137
5	5	134–140	137–148	144–160	5	1	106–118	115–129	125–140
5	6	136–142	139–151	146–164	5	2	108–121	118–132	128–143
5	7	138–145	142–154	149–168	5	3	111–124	121–135	131–147
5	8	140–148	145–157	152–172	5	4	114–127	124–138	134–151
5	9	142–151	148–160	155–176	5	5	117–130	127–141	137–155
5	10	144–154	151–163	158–180	5	6	120–133	130–144	140–159
5	11	146–157	154–166	161–184	5	7	123–136	133–147	143–163
6	0	149–160	157–170	164–188	5	8	126–139	136–150	146–167
6	1	152–164	160–174	168–192	5	9	129–142	139–153	149–170
6	2	155–168	164–178	172–197	5	10	132–145	142–156	152–173
6	3	158–172	167–182	176–202	5	11	135–148	145–159	155–176
6	4	162–176	171–187	181–207	6	0	138–151	148–162	158–179

Note: Weights at ages 25–59 based on lowest mortality. Weight in pounds according to frame (in indoor clothing weighing 5 lbs. for men and 3 lbs. for women; shoes with 1″ heels).

Source: Society of Actuaries, and Association of Life Insurance Medical Directors of America, *1979 Build Study,* 1980.

Weight charts, such as the 1983 Metropolitan Height and Weight Tables shown here, are helpful in determining desirable weight. We can't change our basic body structure, but we can work at becoming more fit than fat.

calories, without increasing physical activity, an approach that is unlikely to have lasting results. Besides the calories burned during exercise, there is a second, perhaps more important, reason to include physical activity in any weight-loss regimen. Following exercise, the body's metabolic rate is stimulated so that additional calories are burned afterwards for several hours (4). This increased calorie-burning efficiency *after* exercise is a great aid to losing weight and keeping it off. Exercise also helps prevent loss of muscle as pounds are lost.

Many people can, in fact, lose their excess fat simply by

(continued on p. 54)

What *Is* a Gram of Fat . . . and How Many Should You Eat?

Complete the following sentences.

1. A gram is a unit of *(a)* weight *(b)* size *(c)* energy

2. One gram of fat contains *(a)* 4 calories *(b)* 9 calories *(c)* 14 calories

3. If a product has 100 calories and 4 grams of fat, the percentage of calories that come from fat is *(a)* 40 *(b)* 4 *(c)* 36

4. If a woman eats 1,600 calories a day and wants to make sure she is following the recommendation of the American Heart Association and the National Cancer Institute to take in no more than 30 percent of her calories as fat, the number of grams of fat she should consume daily amounts to a maximum of *(a)* 43 *(b)* 53 *(c)* 63

Confused? If the answer is "yes," you're not alone. So are the vast majority of Americans, even though most newspaper and magazine articles that advise consumers on how to cut down on fat mention *grams* and every food with a nutrition label lists the number of grams of fat in a serving.

The problem is that the numbers often appear without any explanation of what they represent. Only rarely is the reader told how to translate the grams of fat in the foods he or she eats into the percentage of calories that come from fat.

Hence this Special Report, wherein we spell out the exact meaning of one gram of fat and why knowing it is invaluable for healthful eating. Moreover, we show you how to calculate just how many grams of fat you can eat in a day without going over the limit of 30 percent of total calories recommended by most major health organizations.

These aides to a reduced-fat lifestyle concern you—or someone you know. More than a third of all Americans aged 20 to 74—some 60 million people—have high blood cholesterol levels according to a major study released by government researchers. And dietary modification, they say, should be the primary mode of treatment for this condition, which can contribute to heart disease.

Lowering blood cholesterol is not the only benefit derived from eating less fat, however. It can be the answer to previously unsuccessful attempts at weight loss, perhaps ward off certain cancers such as cancer of the breast and colon, and play a role in lowering high blood pressure. Fortunately, following a lower-fat plan is much less punishing than trading in beef for bean sprouts, as you will see. But first, some basics.

The fat facts that usually go unexplained

Imagine holding two very tiny pieces of coal, one in each hand. Their weights are exactly the same, a twenty-eighth of an ounce or one gram. But one is able to give off more heat than the other. That's because it has more heat-producing energy; that is, calories. When it burns, it releases 9 calories of energy, but the other yields less than half that amount—just 4 calories. That's how it is with fat, carbohydrate, and protein.

Each gram of fat contains 9 calories, whereas the same weight of carbohydrate or protein provides only 4, which is why fat is more "fattening" than protein or carbohydrate. But how do these differences work when it comes to the fat in foods? A comparison of whole milk, 2% fat milk, 1% fat milk, and skim milk provides some ready answers. One cup of any of these milks *weighs* the same amount—about 244 grams or some 8.5 ounces. With whole milk, 8 of those grams— about 3.25 percent of the total—come from fat. Thus, technically speaking, whole milk could be called 3.25% fat. But since gram for gram, fat has more than twice the calories of carbohydrate or protein, some math is in order to see what percentage is fat in terms of *calories* rather than weight.

The first step is to find out how many calories are in a cup of whole milk. The fat itself contributes 72 calories (8 grams × 9 calories per gram

= 72). Carbohydrate, which makes up 11 of the grams, provides 44 calories (11 grams × 4 calories per gram = 44). The 8 grams of protein present supply 32 calories (8 grams × 4 calories per gram = 32). And the water in milk—the lion's share of its weight at over 200 grams—has no calories whatsoever, making the total calorie count 148 or, for convenience's sake, 150 (72 + 44 + 32 = 148). The next step, determining the percentage of the total 150 calories that come from fat, requires only a simple calculation. Just multiply the 72 calories of fat by 100 for a figure of 7,200 and then divide by the 150-calorie total for a result of 48 (72 × 100/150 = 48). What it means is that while the product is only 3.25 percent fat by weight, it amounts to 48 percent fat by calories and is a much fattier food than it seems at first glance.

How much of the food is fat

To figure out the percentage of calories in a food that come from fat

1. *Multiply the number of grams of fat in the food by 9.*

2. *Multiply the answer in step one by 100.*

3. *Divide the outcome of step two by the total number of calories in the product.*

As for 2% fat milk, one cup contains 120 calories and 5 grams of fat. In other words, those 5 grams make up only 2 percent of the milk's 244-gram weight, but as you probably already suspect the story is much different caloriewise. The 5 grams contribute 45 calories (5 × 9) or 38 percent of the 120-calorie total (45 × 100/120 = 38).

When it comes to 1 % milk, only 2 grams of fat can be found in a cup. But since those 2 grams have 18 calories (2 × 9) and the milk has just 100 calories altogether, fat makes up 18 percent of the calorie count (18 × 100/100 = 18).

Skim milk has less than a gram of fat or, for all practical purposes, no grams of fat whatsoever. Thus, none of its 90 calories come from fat.

The milk figures may make it seem as though someone who is trying to follow a diet that gets no more than 30 percent of its calories from fat can never drink whole or 2% fat milk, because the first is 48 percent fat calories and the other is 38 percent. But it doesn't work that way. Granted, fitting high-fat foods into a reduced-fat diet requires some thought, but all the foods eaten in a day need to be looked at together.

Some, such as margarine and the oil used in cooking and on salads, get 100 percent of their calories from fat, since fat is their only calorie-containing ingredient. Fruits and vegetables, on the other hand, have hardly any fat at all. Thus, if a health-conscious eater makes sure to eat plenty of fruits and vegetables and uses oil and margarine sparingly, he or she will have a better chance of averaging out the day's fat calories to less that 30 percent of the total. Similarly, if a person cannot abide anything other than whole milk or even higher-fat cream in his two daily cups of coffee, he can make prudent choices with other foods that will allow him that indulgence and still stay within the low-fat guidelines.

Even entire days of high-fat eating now and then can fit into a normally low-fat diet as long as they remain the exception rather than become the rule. If that were not the case, holidays like Thanksgiving and Christmas would be out the window. But how, you may ask, is one to keep track? Nobody's mind works in such computer-like fashion that he or she can constantly be adding up the grams in every single food that is eaten, figuring out the percentage of calories that come from fat in each item, and averaging out those percentages throughout the day or over the course of several days. Don't worry; nobody's mind needs to. There's a shortcut.

A simple gram count is all it takes

To make sure that no more than 30 percent of total calories come from fat, all anyone needs to do is figure out the average number of calories in the foods eaten daily, take 30 percent of that average, and then divide by 9 to determine how many grams of fat will squeeze into the particular figure arrived at.

simply as a matter of principle but now realizes it's something she's going to have to get serious about; she has just gone for her first physical in many years and learned that she has high blood cholesterol. Carol is at an advantage since, as an on-again, off-again dieter, she has learned the approximate number of calories in most of the items she eats and already knows that she takes in about 1,800 calories a day. her next step is to figure out 30 percent of 1,800, which is accomplished by multiplying 1,800 by .30 for a total of 540. In other words, she has 540 calories a day to "spend" on fat. The question now become how many grams of fat can "fit" into 540 calories. Since each gram comes to 9 calories, all she has to do is divide 540 by 9 for a total of 60 grams.

The formula becomes clearer with an example. Take 39-year-old Carol. She has been trying in a casual way to follow a low-fat diet for some time

Easy ways to cut fat from your diet

To make reducing your fat intake not just simple but also relatively painless

Switch from	to	Fat savings
2 tbsp fudge topping	2 tbsp chocolate syrup	4 grams
1 slice French Toast	4″ pancake	5 grams
Snickers Bar	Three Musketeers Bar	5 grams
3 oz chicken breast & skin	3 oz skinless chicken breast	4 grams
1 large egg	1/4 cup Egg Beaters	5 grams
1 slice Oscar Mayer bologna	1 slice Oscar Mayer 95% Fat Free Smoked Cooked Ham	3 grams
3 oz breaded, fried shrimp	3 oz boiled shrimp	9 grams
Ramen Pride Oriental Noodles & Pork Flavor soup, 10 oz	Campbell's Chicken Noodle soup	6 grams

Answers to opening quiz: 1. (a); 2. (b); 3. (c); 4. (b)

Source: *Tufts University Diet & Nutrition Letter,* Vol. 7, No. 8, October 1989, pp. 3, 6.

increasing physical activity (aerobic activity in particular such as brisk walking, jogging, aerobic dance, rowing, cycling). Others will need to combine a moderate reduction in caloric intake (250–500 calories) with regular physical activity. A weight-reduction plan should, at a minimum, include the servings specified in the Daily Food Guide (see chapter 2); supply adequate protein and carbohydrates; and be low in fat, added sugars, and alcohol, which provide concentrated calories.

If food intake is reduced, a caution is in order. Cutting calories can be taken too far, and actually make it easy to regain fat. This sounds paradoxical! But researchers have found that when fewer calories than the metabolic rate requires are consumed, the body compensates by slowing its metabolic rate to conserve energy (5). This means fewer calories are burned and weight loss becomes difficult.

In addition, a too-low calorie level stimulates the body to break down and burn lean muscle tissue to provide needed fuel. Although some fat is burned, it is far less than muscle. As much as two-thirds of the weight lost on a crash diet or very low-calorie diet is muscle and water. As the proportion of muscle to fat in the body decreases, one becomes "fatter" on the inside even though the scale indicates a loss of pounds. This shift causes the metabolic rate to slow further. Weight loss becomes even more difficult but regaining lost weight (which goes back on as fat!) becomes all too easy (5).

We started out by saying that to lose weight, one can either take in fewer calories or expend more calories. Exercise is one obvious way to expend calories, but keeping one's metabolic rate high (and therefore one's calorie-burning ability) is equally important. To do this one must both be physically active and consume at least the number of calories the metabolic rate requires. From this discussion three rules of thumb for weight loss arise:

1. Exercise, exercise, exercise.

2. Don't overeat.

3. Don't severely undereat.

Dietitians and nutritionists involved in weight management programs often recommend women not consume less than 1200 calories a day and men not consume less than 1500 calories. This helps prevent the metabolic rate from slowing and should result in a loss of one-half to 2 pounds a week, a rate considered optimal for ensuring that fat, not muscle, is lost and that the weight will stay off.

Underweight

Being physically fit equates with health, but being extremely thin does not. In addition to the likelihood of poor nutritional health, there is evidence that below-average body weight is associated with long-term problems just as is being overweight. The Framingham heart study found that people with lower body weights were more likely to develop heart disease than those whose weight was average (6).

(continued on p. 57)

Did You Know That . . .
To Approximate Your Frame Size . . .

Extend your arm and bend the forearm upward at a 90 degree angle. Keep fingers straight and turn the inside of your wrist toward your body. Place thumb and index finger of your other hand on the two prominent bones on either side of your elbow. Measure the space between your fingers against a ruler or tape measure. Compare it with these tables that list elbow measurements for medium-framed men and women. Measurements lower than those listed indicate you have a small frame.

Height in 1" heels Men	Elbow Breadth
5' 2"–5' 3"	$2^1/_2"$–$2^7/_8"$
5' 4"–5' 7"	$2^5/_8"$–$2^7/_8"$
5' 8"–5' 11"	$2^3/_4$–3"
6' 0"–6' 3"	$2^3/_4"$–$3^1/_8"$
6' 4"	$2^7/_8"$–$3^1/_4"$

Women	
4' 10"–4' 11"	$2^1/_4"$–$2^1/_2"$
5' 0"–5' 3"	$2^1/_4"$–$2^1/_2"$
5' 4"–5' 7"	$2^3/_8"$–$2^5/_8"$
5' 8"–5' 11"	$2^3/_8"$–$2^5/_8"$
6' 0"	$2^1/_2"$–$2^3/_4"$

First the bad news or, at least, news that is not as good as you may have thought. Exercise does not, as some reports suggest, increase the number of calories burned by the body for 48 hours after the activity ends. Researchers are now saying that it is only up to 12 hours after vigorous physical activity comes to a halt that the body burns extra calories. The reason: Exercise causes a rise in the resting metabolic rate—the rate at which calories are used for normal body functions such as breathing—for a maximum of only half a day, not two days. Interestingly, the effect

Exercise Burns Calories in More Ways than One

appears greater for people who have just begun an exercise program than for those who have been at it for a while. But once an exerciser become more fit and the initial calorie-burning benefit of a quickened metabolism drops off, others kick in.

One has to do with the fact that muscle burns more calories than fat does. It works like this: the more exercise someone engages in, the more muscle he will build up and the more fat he will lose, so his body will burn more calories to maintain itself than it did formerly.

Just as becoming proportionately leaner can raise the number of calories used, so can increased fitness itself, although researchers are not yet sure why that happens. They are sure, however, that the number of calories needed to digest food and store nutrients, called the thermic effect of feeding, rises along with the resting metabolic rate in a just-exercised body. That's especially true for people who are already lean and fit. In fact, as an individual increases his level of fitness, the thermic effect of feeding is raised in response to meals eaten even many hours after an exercise session. (In obese people, the thermic effect of feeding is blunted.)

Exercise provides an added bonus when used in conjunction with caloric restriction through dieting. How? When a person eats less in an effort to drop pounds, his body perceives itself to be in a state of starvation and tries to hold onto calories by decreasing the resting metabolic rate and the thermic effect of feeding. But moderate exercise *combined* with caloric restriction can overturn or at least retard the metabolic slowdown.

Individually, each effect is relatively small in relation to total daily caloric use. However, taken together, these components of what scientists call adaptive thermogenesis can account for as much as 5 to 7 percent of a person's calorie burning, or somewhere in the neighborhood of 100 calories a day. Over the course of a year, that could mean five to 10 pounds to someone trying to shed excess weight. And that's on top of any pounds taken off via the calorie expenditure involved in the exercise itself.

Source: *Tufts University Diet & Nutrition Letter,* Vol. 7, No. 10, December 1989.

Gaining weight can be as hard for the underweight person as losing weight is for the overweight. High-calorie foods, frequent meals and snacks, and patience are often required. When excessive physical activity is a factor, exercise may need to be reduced until a fit body weight is attained.

The emphasis our culture places on being slim has led to an unprecedented concern about body weight and fear of fat. As many as 50 percent of women of normal weight report they feel too fat (7). Anxiety over body weight and food intake has led to an increase in the eating disorders anorexia nervosa (willful starvation) and bulimia (the binge-purge syndrome). The disorders are complex in origin and treatment requires both psychological and nutritional counseling.

For an in-depth look at overweight, underweight, and eating disorders, see the book in this series, Wellness: Weight Control.

In Summary

Eating according to one's appetite, consuming a varied, nutrient-rich diet with reasonable levels of fat and sugar, and engaging in regular physical activity keep the body in energy balance, where weight is neither gained nor lost. For those who need to lose body fat, a low-fat diet with a moderate reduction in calories combined with increased physical activity leads to feeling well and looking good, and allows the body to reach and maintain a healthy, fit weight without the need for crash dieting, rigid calorie counting, or undue anxiety about every bite of food that goes in the mouth. Eat well, be active, and enjoy!

CARBOHYDRATES: THE REAL FOOD OF CHAMPIONS

Carbohydrates make up the largest portion of most diets. These organic plant compounds are the starches, sugars, and fibers in our food. Starches, also called complex carbohydrates, are made of long chains of sugar molecules (specifically, the sugar molecule **glucose**) linked together like beads in a necklace. Once digested and absorbed, the glucose molecules, now separated, travel in the blood and are used to fuel body cells. Complex carbohydrates are abundant in grains, breads, potatoes, winter squash, carrots, peas, corn, and dry beans and peas. Other vegetables and fruits provide lesser amounts.

Glucose: A monosaccharide or simple sugar found in foods by itself and also as part of complex carbohydrates and the disaccharides sucrose, maltose, and lactose; also known as blood sugar.

(continued on p. 60)

Kudos for women. More and more are heeding the advice to reduce the fat in their diets. Over the course of an average three days' worth of eating, 43 percent fewer women consumed high-fat cuts of beef and pork in 1985 than did the women of almost a decade earlier. In addition, 11 percent fewer drank whole milk, and 18 percent more drank two or one percent fat milk as well as skim milk. Furthermore, the women were less likely to eat chicken that had been fried or still had the skin on.

What Women Are Eating

[R]esults reflect major healthful changes in the way women are now eating, say researchers at the University of North Carolina who compared the eating patterns of 5,400 women in 1977–78 with the dietary habits of more than 1,000 women eight years later. They also observed that the more education women receive, the more likely they are to make healthful eating choices, which suggests that they are particularly adept at absorbing nutrition information and "translating" it appropriately.

Unfortunately, the scientists did come across some less-than-favorable shifts. Some 12 percent more women ate high-fat cheeses in 1985 than in 1977–78. More women also ate potato, corn, and tortilla chips as well as buttered popcorn. And they indulged more heavily in ice cream, cakes, cookies, pies, doughnuts, and granola bars.

Those alterations could reflect a "yuppie diet," speculates Barry Popkin, PhD, professor of nutrition at the University of North Carolina. Women may exercise a lot and then splurge on fatty desserts and snack foods later, he explains. Or, he says, the changes could be due to the fact that women have more choices today than they had 10 years ago and are eating away from home and snacking more often. That hypothesis seems particularly plausible in light of another recent study of women's diets, which suggests the greater the extent of their dining out, the higher the amount of saturated as well as total fat they consume for every 1,000 calories eaten, not to mention the lower their intake of iron, calcium, vitamin C, carbohydrate, and fiber.

Nevertheless, Dr. Popkin says, it does appear that old patterns of eating are changing, and the not-so-healthful modifications are not altogether undoing the overall positive trend. In 1977, women took in an average of 42 percent of total calories from fat according to the U.S. Department of Agriculture. In 1985, that number dropped to 38 percent—still quite a distance from the recommended 30 percent goal, but certainly a move in the right direction.

Source: *Tufts University Diet & Nutrition Letter,* Vol. 7, No. 10, December 1989.

Little Things Add Up

It's easier to incorporate small switches and substitutions in your eating habits than to initiate radical changes. These simple suggestions for a more healthful diet can reduce your fat, calories, and cholesterol intake considerably while still satisfying your appetite. To put these number in perspective, if you consume 2,000 calories a day, you should eat no more than about 66 grams of fat—that way fat will contribute less than 30% of your daily calories.

INSTEAD OF EATING	SUBSTITUTE	TO SAVE*
1 croissant	1 plain bagel	35 calories, 10 grams fat, 13 mg cholesterol
1 cup cooked egg noodles	1 cup cooked macaroni	50 milligrams cholesterol
1 whole egg	1 egg white	65 calories, 6 grams fat, 220 mg cholesterol
1 oz Cheddar cheese	1 oz part-skim mozzarella	35 calories, 4 grams fat, 15 mg cholesterol
1 oz cream cheese	1 oz cottage cheese (1% fat)	74 calories, 9 grams fat, 29 mg cholesterol
1 tbsp whipping cream	1 tbsp evaporated skim milk, whipped	32 calories, 5 grams fat
3.5 oz skinless roast duck	3.5 oz skinless roast chicken	46 calories, 7 grams fat
3.5 oz beef tenderloin, choice, untrimmed, broiled	3.5 oz beef tenderloin, select, trimmed, broiled	75 calories, 10 grams fat
3.5 oz lamb chop, untrimmed, broiled	3.5 oz lean leg of lamb, trimmed, broiled	219 calories, 28 grams fat
3.5 oz pork spare ribs, cooked	3.5 oz lean pork loin, trimmed, broiled	157 calories, 17 grams fat
1 oz regular bacon, cooked	1 oz Canadian bacon, cooked	111 calories, 12 grams fat
1 oz hard salami	1 oz extra-lean roasted ham	75 calories, 8 grams fat
1 beef frankfurter	1 chicken frankfurter	67 calories, 8 grams fat
3 oz oil-packed tuna, light	3 oz water-packed tuna, light	60 calories, 6 grams fat
1 regular-size serving fast-food French fries	1 medium-sized baked potato	125 calories, 11 grams fat
1 oz oil-roasted peanuts	1 oz roasted chestnuts	96 calories, 13 grams fat
1 oz potato chips	1 oz thin pretzels	40 calories, 9 grams fat
1 oz corn chips	1 oz plain air-popped popcorn	125 calories, 9 grams fat
1 tbsp sour-cream dip	1 tbsp bottled salsa	20 calories, 3 grams fat
1 glazed doughnut	1 slice angel-food cake	110 calories, 13 grams fat, 21 mg cholesterol
3 chocolate sandwich cookies	3 fig bar cookies	4 grams fat
1 oz unsweetened chocolate	3 tbsp cocoa powder	73 calories, 13 grams fat
1 cup ice cream (premium)	1 cup sorbet	320 calories, 34 grams fat, 100 mg cholesterol

*The values listed are the most significant savings; smaller differences are not shown. Weights given for meats are edible portions.

Source: *University of California Berkeley Wellness Letter,* Vol. 5, No. 12, September 1989, p. 3.

Table 3.2 Approximate Carbohydrate Content of Foods

Food	Carbohydrate (grams)
1 slice bread	
¹/₂ cup cooked cereal or grain or pasta	
1 tortilla	
¹/₂ english muffin	
¹/₂ bagel	15
1 dinner roll	
¹/₃ to ¹/₂ cup white potato, corn, lima beans, peas	
6 saltines	
¹/₂ cup cooked legumes (dried beans and peas)	
¹/₂ cup cooked vegetables	
1 cup raw vegetables	5
¹/₂ cup fruit or juice	
¹/₂ banana	
1 small apple or orange	
12 grapes	10
¹/₄ cantaloupe melon	
¹/₂ grapefruit	
1 cup milk or plain yogurt	
8 oz. soybean curd (tofu)	12
1 tsp. sugar, honey, jelly	5
1 cupcake with icing	28
1 cup ice cream	27
1 chocolate chip cookie (2 in.)	7

Source: U.S. Dietary Exchange Lists of the American Diabetic Association and USDA Agriculture Handbook No. 456: Nutritive Value of Foods.

While carbohydrates make up the largest portion of most diets, most Americans still need to increase their carbohydrate consumption. Complex carbohydrates (starches) are particularly abundant in grains, breads, potatoes, winter squash, carrots, peas, corn, and dry beans and peas. However, other vegetables and fruits are also useful carbohydrate sources.

Fructose: A monosaccharide or simple sugar, often referred to as fruit sugar. It is also found in honey and is part of the disaccharide sucrose, or table sugar.

Galactose: A monosaccharide or simple sugar; part of the disaccharide lactose found in milk.

Sucrose: A dissaccharide, or sugar composed of two component sugar molecules, glucose and fructose, found in table sugar, beet sugar, and cane sugar.

While starches are large molecules, dietary sugars are small. Three sugar molecules—glucose (the same sugar in starch), **fructose**, and **galactose** either alone or in combination are called the simple carbohydrates or dietary sugars. Table sugar consists of **sucrose** (a glucose molecule linked to a fructose molecule). Honey

Carbohydrates Are Low in Calories!

8 ounce sirloin steak:	880 calories
Baked potato with 2 tsp butter and 2 tbs sour cream:	215 calories

You can eat 4 baked potatoes with butter and sour cream before you consume the same number of calories as the steak!

Source: U.S. Department of Agriculture, *Nutritive Value of American Foods in Common Units*, Handbook No. 456, 1975.

consists mainly of free-floating glucose and fructose molecules. Fruits contain fructose, and milk contains lactose (a glucose molecule and a galactose molecule linked). Once absorbed, both fructose and galactose are converted into glucose, carried in the blood, and used to fuel body cells just as the glucose in starches is. Concentrated sources of sugars include table sugar, honey, molasses, corn syrup, high-fructose corn syrup, pancake syrup, powdered fructose, and brown sugar.

Functions of Carbohydrates

Carbohydrates are essential nutrients because of their role in providing fuel to all body cells. Carbohydrates, in fact, are considered the ideal fuel because unlike protein, fat, and alcohol, they "burn clean," leaving no residue the body must dismantle or excrete. Carbohydrates are the only fuel used by the brain and central nervous system under normal conditions. Because our nerves depend on carbohydrates for their energy supply, they let us know if they are "on empty" through feelings of fatigue, irritability, depression, and lessened ability to concentrate.

Not only nerves, but muscles need carbohydrates as well. A diet high in carbohydrates ensures that muscles, including the heart, have the necessary fuel for physical activity. Some of the carbohydrates not needed immediately after a meal are stored in liver and muscle cells as a compound called **glycogen**. The more glycogen stored and available as fuel in the muscles and liver, the longer one can run or swim or work. For this reason, endurance athletes such as long-distance runners perform best when their diet is high in carbohydrates.

Glycogen: A form of complex carbohydrate stored in the body. It is found primarily in liver and muscle tissue.

How Much Carbohydrate?

It surprises many people that carbohydrates should be the largest component of a healthy diet, providing at least 55 percent of calories. For years, the myth has abounded that starches or complex carbohydrates are fattening or unhealthy foods, although they are quite moderate in calories and often rich in nutrients.

Table 3.3 Carbohydrate Comparison Diets

Diet Low in Carbohydrate	Diet High in Carbohydrate
2 slices whole wheat toast	3 whole wheat pancakes
2 tsp butter or margarine	2 tsp butter or margarine
2 eggs, fried	$1/2$ cup applesauce
Coffee w/1 tsp sugar	1 cup skim milk
	$3/4$ cup orange juice
2 beef tacos	Bean burrito
12 oz. soft drink	$3/4$ cup mixed fruit
	1 cup skim milk
2 oz peanuts	Bagel w/2 tbs apple butter
	Pear
Baked chicken breast	Baked chicken breast
$1/2$ cup mashed potatoes	$3/4$ cup mashed potatoes
1 tsp butter or margarine	2 tsp butter or margarine
$1/2$ cup green beans	$1/2$ cup green beans
1 cup green salad	1 cup salad
2 tbs salad dressing	2 tbs salad dressing
7 oz wine	2 dinner rolls
	7 oz wine
Total Calories: Approximately 2000	**Total Calories: Approximately 2000**
Grams of carbohydrate: 141	**Grams of carbohydrate: 287**
Percent carbohydrate: 28%	**Percent carbohydrate: 57%**

Source: Adapted from American Diabetic Association and American Dietetic Association, *Exchange Lists for Meal Planning.*

If, like most Americans, your diet contains too much fat and too few carbohydrates, one relatively simple route to a more balanced diet is to substitute foods high in complex carbohydrates for those high in fat.

For example, an 8-ounce steak provides 800 calories, while the baked potato that goes with it provides only 80 calories. A slice of bread provides about the same number of calories as an apple. Ten slices of bread yield 700 calories, only one-third of the calories needed daily by the average woman. So, carbohydrates do not cause weight gain in and of themselves. But excess calories from any source (whether carbohydrates, proteins, fats, or alcohol) can be changed into fat and stored as fat tissue.

Approximately 100 grams of carbohydrate a day is considered a minimum nutritional requirement (the amount in 5 slices of bread, an apple, and a glass of milk, for example) (8). For optimal health, more than this is needed. About 220 to 300 grams will be needed by most people to achieve the currently recommended 55 percent carbohydrate level (menus low and high in carbohydrates are shown in table 3.3).

Because the American diet tends to be too high in fat, substituting additional complex carbohydrate foods for high-fat foods helps the diet become more balanced in both respects. Current dietary guidelines suggest we eat at least 6 servings daily of breads, cereals, and legumes and 5 servings of a combination of fruits and vegetables (9).

Whole Grains and Refined Grains

Major shifts have occurred in the type of breads and grains consumed in this country during the last century. Prior to the 1930s, most bread was made from whole wheat and other unrefined grains. By the 1940s, bread made from refined white flour had virtually replaced whole wheat bread.

Because many nutrients are lost when the bran and germ of the whole wheat kernel are removed to make white flour, a law was passed in the 1940s requiring refined white flour to be enriched with nutrients in order to prevent nutrient deficiencies. Three B vitamins (niacin, riboflavin, and thiamin) and the mineral iron are now added back into white flour. But over a dozen additional vitamins, trace minerals, and fiber are still missing from the refined product. The box on page 66 shows the difference in several nutrients between enriched wheat bread and whole wheat bread.

As nutritional science has progressed, awareness has grown that these missing nutrients and fiber are important to health and are sometimes marginally low in the diet. For example, chromium is a trace mineral lost in refining that is essential to glucose metabolism and its deficiency may be a factor in the development of diabetes in adults (10, 11). Fiber and nutrient losses also occur when brown rice is refined to white rice and

(continued on p. 65)

For whole-wheat bread to be 100 percent whole-wheat, the first ingredient listed on the label must be whole-wheat flour. If additional flours are listed, or words like "wheat" or "cracked wheat" appear on the label, then the bread usually contains processed white flour.

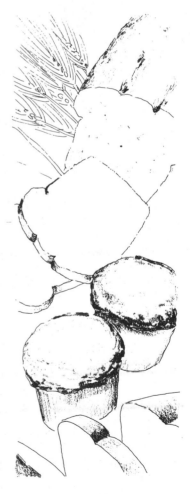

A Pattern for Daily Food Choices

When shopping, planning, and preparing meals for yourself and others, use this guide for a varied and nutritious diet . . .

- Choose foods daily from each of the first five major groups shown below.
- Include different foods from within the groups. As a guide, you can use the subgroups listed below the major food group heading.
- Have at least the minimum number of servings suggested from each group. Limit total amount of food eaten to maintain desirable body weight.
- For most people, choose foods that are low in fat and sugars more often.
- Go easy on fats, sweets, and alcoholic beverages.

Food group	Suggested daily servings
Breads, cereals, and other grain products Whole-grain Enriched	6 to 11 (Include several servings a day of whole-grain products)
Fruit Citrus, melon, berries Other fruit	2 to 4
Vegetables Dark-green leafy Deep yellow Dry beans and peas (legumes) Starchy Other vegetables	3 to 5 servings (Include all types regularly; use dark-green leafy vegetables and dry beans and peas several times a week)
Meat, poultry, fish, and alternates (Eggs, dry beans and peas, nuts, and seeds)	2 to 3 servings—total 5 to 7 ounces lean

Milk, cheese, and yogurt	2–3 servings for men 3–4 servings for women 2 or more servings for children 4 servings for teens and women who are pregnant or breastfeeding
Fats, sweets, and alcoholic beverages	Avoid too many fats and sweets. If you drink alcoholic beverages, do so in moderation.

*NOTE: The pattern for daily food choices described here was developed for Americans who regularly eat foods from all the major food groups listed. Some people, such as vegetarians and others, may not eat one or more of these types of foods. These people may wish to contact a registered dietitian (RD) in their community for help in planning food choices.

Source: *Adapted from United States Department of Agriculture Nutrition Information Services, *Home & Garden Bulletin* No. 232–1.

WHAT COUNTS AS A SERVING?

The examples listed below will give you an idea of the amounts of food to count as one serving when you use the guide to the left.

Breads, cereals, and other grain products: 1 slice of· bread, $1/2$ hamburger bun or English muffin, a small roll, biscuit, or muffin; 3 to 4 small or 2 large crackers; $1/2$ cup cooked cereal, rice, or pastas, or 1 ounce of ready-to-eat breakfast cereal.

Fruit: A piece of whole fruit, such as an apple, banana, orange, a grapefruit half, or a melon wedge; $3/4$ cup of juice, $1/2$ cup berries, or $1/2$ cup cooked or canned fruit; or $1/4$ cup dried fruit.

Vegetables: $1/2$ cup of cooked or chopped raw vegetables or 1 cup of leafy raw vegetables, such as lettuce or spinach.

Meat, poultry, fish, and alternates: Serving sizes will differ. Amounts should total 5 to 7 ounces of lean meat, fish, or poultry a day. A serving of meat the size and thickness of the palm of a woman's hand is about 3 to 5 ounces and a man's, 5 to 7 ounces. Count 1 egg, $1/2$ cup cooked dry beans, or 2 tablespoons of peanut butter as 1 ounce of lean meat.

Milk, cheese, and yogurt: 1 cup of milk, 8 ounces of yogurt, 1½ ounces natural cheese, or 2 ounces of process cheese.

WHAT ABOUT THE NUMBER OF SERVINGS?
The amount of food you need depends on your age, sex, physical condition, and how active you are. Almost everyone should have at least the minimum number of servings from each food group daily. Many women, older children, and most teenagers and men need more. The top of the range is about right for an active man or teenage boy. Young children may not need as much food; they can have smaller servings from all groups except milk, which should total 2 servings per day. You can use the guide at the left to help plan for the variety and amounts of foods your family needs each day.

Source: *The Dietary Guidelines: Seven Ways to Help Yourself to Good Health and Nutrition,* The American Dietetic Association, Chicago, 1987.

---

whole cornmeal to refined, degermed cornmeal. Thus, making whole grain choices is an important part of a nutritious eating plan. The benefits of consuming whole grains for their fiber content is discussed on page 73.

Sweet Facts
Although sugar has received its share of bad press in recent years, small amounts of sugar in the diet appear to pose no health problem. Too many sugary foods, however, can crowd more nutritious foods from the diet, contribute to poor dental health, and add extra fat—all reasons to limit their intake.

Is honey any healthier than table sugar? Although technically honey contains more nutrients than white sugar, the difference is so slight that for practical purposes both sweeteners can be considered empty calorie foods—they provide calories but no additional nutritional value. Honey may be enjoyed for its taste, but not because it has any nutritional benefits.

In the United States, sugar consumption has risen to an average 130 pounds per person per year, or approximately 40 teaspoons a day (12). Refined sugar provided only one-third of the carbohydrates in the average diet of 1910. Today, sugar provides approximately half of the carbohydrates (13).

The Dietary Guidelines for Americans recommend that sugar intake be limited through the following steps (14):

1. Use less of all sugars, including white and brown sugars, raw sugars, honey, and syrups.

Did You Know That . . .

All the calories from hard candy, jelly beans, and regular sodas come from sugar. In a regular soda you are getting 8 to 12 teaspoons of sugar for every 12 ounces you drink.

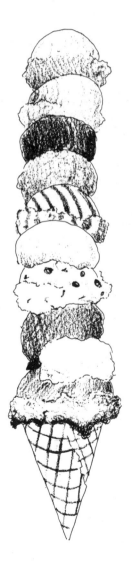

According to the International Association of Ice Cream Manufacturers, enough ice cream is produced each year to provide 10 single-scoop cones for every single person on the planet.

Which Is Better, Enriched White Bread or Whole Wheat?

Compared to whole wheat bread, enriched white bread has only:

4%	of the	vitamin E
12%	of the	manganese
22%	of the	vitamin B6
22%	of the	fiber
28%	of the	chromium
28%	of the	magnesium
38%	of the	potassium
38%	of the	zinc
45%	of the	copper
50%	of the	folacin
56%	of the	pantothenic acid

Source: A. Chenault, *Nutrition and Health* (Holt, Rinehart and Winston, 1984), p. 49.

No one particular food can provide 100 percent of any nutrient, but if we consider that, for the sake of comparison, whole wheat bread provides 100 units of vitamin E, then enriched white bread would provide only 4 units. Thus, whole wheat bread is the more nutritious choice.

2. Eat less of foods containing sugars such as candy, soft drinks, ice cream, cakes, cookies, and pies.

3. Read food labels. If sucrose, glucose, fructose, maltose, dextrose, or lactose appear first on the ingredients list, there is a large amount of sugar in the product.

4. How often we eat sugar is as important as the amount we eat. The more often our teeth are exposed to sugar, the greater the likelihood of dental caries. We should reduce the frequency of foods containing sugar, brush our teeth after eating, and floss regularly.

Although not necessary for health, sugar can be included in the diet at reasonable levels without causing harm. In addition to considering the amount of sugar in desserts, sweets, and beverages, we should be aware that sugar is often "hidden" in other prepared foods. The sugar content of some foods not thought of as being sweet may be a surprise. For example, by weight, nondairy coffee creamer is 65 percent sugar, catsup is 29 percent, bottled salad dressing is 30 percent, and Shake 'n' Bake is 51 percent. The teaspoons of sugar in common foods are shown in table 3.4 on page 71.

(continued on p. 73)

FIGURE 3.2
Rating Your Diet: How Sweet Is It?

Take a look at *your* diet. Check the box that most closely describes your eating habits to see how the foods you choose affect the amount of added sugars in your diet.

How Often Do You:	Less Than Once a Week	1 or 2 Times a Week	3 to 5 Times a Week	Almost Daily
1. Drink soft drinks, sweetened fruit drinks, punches or ades?	☐	☐	☐	☐
2. Choose sweet desserts and snacks, such as cakes, pies, cookies, and ice cream?	☐	☐	☐	☐
3. Use canned or frozen fruits packed in heavy syrup or add sugar to fresh fruit?	☐	☐	☐	☐
4. Eat candy?	☐	☐	☐	☐
5. Add sugar to coffee or tea?	☐	☐	☐	☐
6. Use jam, jelly, or honey on bread or rolls?	☐	☐	☐	☐

How Did You Do?
The more often you choose the items listed above, the higher your diet is likely to be in sugars. However, not all of the items listed contribute the same amount of added sugars.

You may need to cut back on sugar-containing foods, especially those you checked as "3 to 5 times a week" or more. This does not mean eliminating these foods from your diet. You can moderate your intake of sugars by choosing foods that are high in sugar less often, and by eating smaller portions.

Source: Adapted from U.S. Department of Agriculture *Home and Garden Bulletin* No. 232–5, April 1986.

FIGURE 3.3
Sugar Consumption

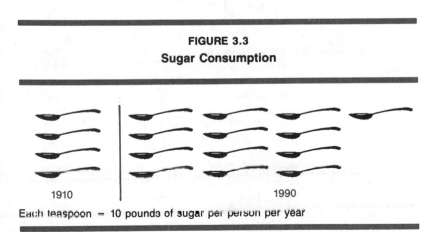

1910   1990

Each teaspoon – 10 pounds of sugar per person per year

The average American's consumption of sugar has more than tripled since the turn of the century. In 1910 average annual consumption was 40 pounds per person. By 1990 it had risen to over 130 pounds.

The Healthy Eater's Guide to Sugar

For many years sugar has had a bad reputation, considered, at the very least, a junk food and an indulgence. More seriously, it has also been said to cause heart disease, obesity, cavities, hyperactivity in children, and diabetes. The quiz below will help you separate the sugar myths from sugar facts.

True or false:

"Sugar" is clearly listed on food labels.
False. It is included in ingredients lists, but usually goes by other names than "sugar." To most people this word means refined, white table sugar (sucrose), made from cane or beets. However, there are actually dozens of sugars: in their pure form they have such names as fructose, glucose (also called dextrose), maltose, lactose, and sugar alcohols like sorbitol and xylitol. Sugars are often identified by their sources, such as maple syrup, honey, corn syrup, and molasses. Any and all of these names may turn up on a label. Obviously, when one of these sugars is listed as the first ingredient in a food, you know that a lot of it was used. But on some food labels, several forms of sugar are listed lower down, and added all together these sugars may be the primary ingredient.

Sugar is, in a sense, the number-one food additive. About 70% of all sweeteners are added by manufacturers to beverages and processed foods for flavor, texture, and sometimes coloring. Sugar turns up in some unlikely places—soups, spaghetti sauces, fruit drinks, frozen dinners, cereals, and yogurts—as well as breads, condiments (a tablespoon of ketchup, for instance, has about a teaspoon of sugar), canned goods, and, of course, soft drinks and what we call "sweets." Sugar also occurs naturally in fruits, vegetables, and dairy products.

Americans are eating less sugar than before.
False. While the amount of refined sugar (sucrose) we eat has dropped since 1975, the total amount of sugars in the typical American diet has remained about the same. That's because there has been a large increase in the use of corn syrup, especially the very sweet and inexpensive high-fructose corn sweetener now used in most sodas and many processed foods.

Each American consumes, on average, about 133 pounds of sugar a year from all sources: that accounts for 20 to 25% of all calories and 500 to 600 calories per day per person.

The body needs sugar.
True. Glucose, the main sugar in the blood and a basic fuel for the body, is essential to the functioning of all cells, particularly brain cells. But you don't need to *eat* any sugar to supply your body with glucose. All you need is *complex carbohydrates,* which are actually large chains of glucose molecules. (In contrast, sugar is called a *simple carbohydrate* because of its chemical structure.) Complex carbohydrates, also known as starches, are found in foods derived from plants—grains, vegetables, and fruits. In some circumstances, glucose can be derived from the breakdown of protein or fat.

When you eat something sugary, it is broken down to the simplest sugars (unless the food's sugars are already in their simplest forms). For instance, during digestion sucrose is broken down into glucose and fructose, which enter the bloodstream through the walls of the small intestine and travel to the body's cells and the liver. With the aid of the hormone insulin, the cells absorb glucose and use it as energy. Some glucose is stored in the liver and muscles in the form of glycogen; the glycogen in the liver can be readily reconverted to glucose when energy is needed. Most of the fructose is also converted to glucose by the liver. The liver can also convert sugar into some of the building blocks of protein, amino acids. Any excess sugar, like any extra calories, is converted into fat and stored.

Kids have more cavities than ever because they eat so much refined sugar.
False. Half of all children in the U.S. today have *no* cavities at all, though they're eating as much, or more, sugar than ever. Just eating sugar isn't enough to cause cavities. Many factors play a role in tooth decay—including the strength of tooth enamel, which has been greatly improved by long-term fluoridation of most of America's water supply. In any case, while refined sugar remains the leading dietary cause to tooth decay, it is not the only food that promotes cavities. Sugars such as fructose in fruit and lactose in milk may promote decay, as may some foods high in fermentable carbohydrates, such as bread and rice. Other variables also affect tooth decay: the consistency of the food, how long the food remains on the teeth and, of course, how well you clean your teeth.

Sugar is the leading cause of obesity.
False. Basically, eating more calories than you burn up adds pounds to the body—and for most people the lion's share of excess calories come from eating too much fat, not sugar. So concluded two studies last year in the *American Journal of Clinical Nutrition,* which found, surprisingly, that lean people tend to eat more sugar and less fat than obese people. Not only does fat have more calories than sugar (about 36 vs. 16 calories per teaspoon), but studies have also suggested that dietary fat may be more efficiently converted to body fat than carbohydrates are.

People often blame sugary foods for weight gain, forgetting that the cakes, ice cream, chocolate, and cookies they're eating derive most of their calories from fat, not sugar. Many a "sweet tooth" may actually be a "fat tooth." This doesn't mean you won't gain weight if you add sugary snacks to your diet. But it's calories, not sugar, that cause weight gain, and fat provides far more of the calories in the American diet than sugar does.

Artificial sweeteners will make you lose weight.
False. Studies have failed to show that artificial sweeteners keep people from gaining weight, much less help them lose significant amounts. One problem is that instead of eating artificially sweetened foods *in place of* high-calorie ones, many people simply add them to their diet. Also, artificial sweeteners don't suppress appetite—and may even increase it.

Eating too much sugar causes diabetes.
False. This misconception arises because diabetes is characterized by high levels of blood sugar (glucose). Excessive sugar consumption is indeed very dangerous for diabetics, who must curtail their sugar intake. But sugar doesn't cause this disorder. Although obesity is probably the leading risk factor for adult-onset diabetes, sugar is not the major culprit behind most cases of obesity, as we've said. Family history of the disease and advancing age are other important factors.

Hypoglycemia is a common problem.
False. Many people claim to suffer from low blood sugar, or hypoglycemia—and blame it for their fatigue, drowsiness, lightheadedness, or anxiety, for instance—but true hypoglycemia is rare. Long-term hypoglycemia can be life threatening; it isn't a disease, but may be a warning sign of a serious disorder that can disrupt the body's ability to regulate sugar.

When low blood sugar occurs in response to food, it's called reactive hypoglycemia. Normally, however, the liver maintains a relatively constant level of blood sugar. After a meal, blood sugar rises and then returns to normal within two to three hours, as insulin allows the body's cells to utilize it. Some foods—sugary ones as well as some starchy ones—tend to cause a greater rise in insulin, which may result in a rather precipitous drop in blood sugar.

Studies have found that few people with chronic fatigue or restlessness actually have a concurrent drop in blood sugar. Conversely, most people have no adverse symptoms when their blood sugar temporarily dips. Don't automatically blame hypoglycemia for mood swings.

Sugar makes children hyperactive.
False. Though for years parents have been blaming a high sugar intake for their children's uncontrollable behavior, a recent review in the *Annals of Allergy* found no strong evidence for this. A 1988 study at the University of Washington School of Medicine came to the same conclusion.

The jury is still out as to whether there's any consistent cause-and-effect relationship between sugar and behavior. Early investigators reported that eating excessive sweets may lead to aggressive and even criminal behavior in adults. However, some experiments during the past decade have found that a meal high in carbohydrates (whether sugars or starches) and low in protein may lead to a relaxed feeling, sleepiness, and decreased alertness by boosting the level of a brain neurotransmitter called serotonin.

You can become addicted to sugar.
False. There's no evidence for this. People don't become physically dependent on sugar—that is, when they stop eating it they don't experience the physical withdrawal symptoms associated with truly addictive substances. There is a popular belief that refined sugar, like drugs, causes a "high" or "rush"—in this case by boosting blood sugar. Other foods, however, such as bananas or dried fruit, may raise blood sugar just as much, and no one claims they're addictive. It is true that humans have an inborn preference for sweets. This may have evolved as a protective mechanism to ensure that our early ancestors ate enough high-calorie foods or tended to choose nontoxic foods such as fruit. And people do crave pleasurable foods. But this doesn't qualify as an addiction.

Sugar in fruit is good, sugar in candy is bad.
False. The sugar is most fruit is primarily fructose, which has few, if any, advantages over sucrose. Like other sugars, it is converted to glucose in the body.

Fruit actually contains a combination of fructose, sucrose, and glucose. (In fact, sucrose is the main sugar in some fruit, such as oranges, melons, and peaches.) One good thing about getting your sugar from fruit rather than from candy or soda is that it comes with vitamins, minerals, and fiber, while the sugary snacks provide only calories, which are thus sometimes called "empty calories." For instance, a glass of orange juice and a glass of cola contain about the same amount of sugar and number of calories, but the juice is high in vitamin C, beta carotene, and potassium.

In contrast, fruit spreads sweetened with fruit juice concentrate are not significantly lower in calories or higher in nutrients than spreads containing sucrose.

Honey and brown sugar aren't more nutritious.
True. Sugar is sugar, and none offers significant nutritional advantages (except blackstrap molasses, which is rich in iron). Brown sugar is usually white sugar with a little molasses added for coloring and flavor, or else it's sucrose that has been slightly less refined. Honey is a little sweeter than table sugar, but the amounts of additional nutrients in it are minuscule.

Sugar can raise blood cholesterol in most people.
False. Dietary sugar has no such adverse effect in most individuals. A task force of scientists convened by the FDA concluded in 1986 that there was no conclusive evidence that a high-sugar intake is a risk factor for heart disease—whether by raising blood cholesterol, triglycerides (a fat in the blood), or blood pressure—"in the general population."

However, some researchers suggest that a small number of "carbohydrate-sensitive" individuals with insulin or triglyceride levels that are high to start with may be particularly sensitive to sugar (especially fructose) and respond by increasing cholesterol and triglyceride levels.

Eating a candy bar before exercising will give you "quick energy."
False. It's likely to be counterproductive, and

may inhibit athletic performance if eaten *right before* an event. The candy bar indeed raises the glucose level in the blood and thus provides some energy for a short while. In response, however, your body releases insulin, which temporarily drops the glucose level even lower than it was to start. Thus if you eat the candy right before a long workout, it can cause faster exhaustion, since your body has to call on its energy reserves (glycogen) earlier than it normally would. In contrast, complex carbohydrates, in foods such as bread or pasta, are slowly absorbed by the body and thus have a steadier effect on blood sugar.

An exception: consuming a sugary snack or beverage *during a workout lasting longer than two hours* (such as a marathon) may enhance your performance and stave off fatigue by supplying you with additional energy.

It's best to eat as little sugar as possible. False. There's no reason to go so far unless you are diabetic or carbohydrate-sensitive, and even most diabetics are allowed occasional sweets. *The best advice is the USDA's vague admonition to "avoid too much sugar."* The only well-substantiated argument against sugar is that it contributes to dental decay. It's also true that most sweets, with the exception of fruit, are high in fat and calories and low in nutrients. If the cola you're drinking is taking the place of skim milk, it's a bad trade-off. But if you are a eating a balanced diet that's low in fat and high in complex carbohydrates, there's nothing wrong with eating sugar.

Source: *University of California Berkeley Wellness Letter,* Vol. 6, No. 3, December 1989.

TABLE 3.4 How Sweet Is It?

Food (Serving size)	Sugar Calories (% of total calories)	Teaspoons of Added Sugar
Beverages		
Brandy, cognac *(1 oz.)*	41	1.7
Dessert wine *(3.5 oz.)*	35	3.0
Gatorade *(8 oz.)*	100	3.5
Nestea Light *(8 oz.)*	100	3.7
Nestea Iced Tea, sugar *(8 oz.)*	97	5.7
Country Time Lemonade Flavor, concentrate *(8 oz.)*	100	6.0
Canada Dry tonic water *(12 oz.)*	98	8.4
Sprite *(12 oz.)*	100	9.0
Cakes		
Cupcake, no icing *(2¹/₂" dia.)*	28	1.5
Cupcake, w/icing *(2¹/₂" dia.)*	40	3.2
Twinkies *(1)*	47	4.8
Yellow cake, no icing *(2.3 oz.)*	38	4.9
Chocolate cake, no icing *(2.3 oz.)*	39	5.3
Candy		
Mr. Goodbar *(1 oz.)*	28	2.7
Peanut M & M's *(14)*	34	3.0

(continued next page)

Hershey's Milk Chocolate w/Almonds *(1 oz.)*	32	3.2
Nestle's Milk Chocolate w/Almonds *(1 oz.)*	34	3.2
Reese's Peanut Butter Cup *(1.6 oz.)*	28	4.8

Miscellaneous Foods

Skippy Peanut Butter *(2 Tbs.)*	11	1.3
Pork & beans *(1/2 cup)*	25	2.4

Other Desserts & Snacks[1]

Bran muffin *(1.6 oz.)*	17	1.2
Danish pastry *(2.3 oz.)*	9	1.5
Glazed doughnut, cake *(1.5 oz.)*	18	1.8
Popsicle *(1)*	100	4.5
Pumpkin pie *(4.6 oz.)*	21	3.6
Apple pie *(4.6 oz.)*	22	4.9

[1] *A 4.6 oz. serving is 1/7 of a pie.*

Breakfast Cereals [1,2]

Grape Nuts	0	0.0
Cheerios	4	0.3
Rice Chex, Wheat, Corn	7	0.5
Special K	11	0.8
Wheaties	11	0.8
Honey Nut Cheerios	36	2.5
Sugar Frosted Flakes	40	2.8
Froot Loops	47	3.3

[1] *Serving size for all breakfast products listed is one ounce, unless indicated.*
[2] *Figures for cereals include naturally occurring sugar in added fruit such as raisins.*

Condiments

Ketchup *(1 Tbs.)*	63	0.6
Table sugar *(1 tsp.)*	100	1.0
Honey *(1 tsp.)*	100	1.4
Jellies, jams, marmalades *(1/2 Tbs.)*	88	1.5
Maple syrup *(1 Tbs.)*	100	3.3

Cookies[1]

Graham crackers *(2 large)*	25	0.9
Peanut butter cookies *(2)*	21	1.8
Brownies w/nuts *(1 oz.)*	28	2.3
Sugar cookies *(2)*	40	3.0

[1] *Serving size for all cookies is about one ounce.*

Dairy Products

Chocolate milk, 2% fat *(1 cup)*	24	2.7
Vanilla ice cream *(1 cup)*	34	5.8
Dannon lowfat yogurt, fruit *(1 cup)*	37	6.0
Thick shake *(11 oz.)*	44	9.6
Ice cream sundae *(1 cup)*	46	19.0

Fruits

Peaches, light syrup, canned *(1/2 cup)*	50	2.3
Pears, heavy syrup, canned *(1/2 cup)*	59	3.6

Source: Adapted from *How Sweet Is It? CSPI's Sugar Scoreboard,* Center for Science in the Public Interest, Washington, DC, 1985.

While not necessary for health, a reasonable amount of sugar can be consumed without risk of harm. However, most American diets include far more sugar than is desirable. A large proportion of this sugar is often "hidden" in processed foods, as can be seen above.

Fiber

Food fibers (with one exception), are carbohydrate compounds in plants that humans cannot digest and absorb, in contrast to starches and sugars. Unlike cows, we lack the necessary enzymes in our digestive tracts to break fiber apart. The fiber we eat does not provide calories and exits the intestinal tract in the stool basically unchanged.

To make matters confusing, however, there are at least seven categories of dietary fiber, including pectins, gums, mucilages, lignins (the noncarbohydrate fiber), algal polysaccharides, celluloses and hemicelluloses. These fibers have different effects in the digestive tract and are found in different foods. Fruits (especially apples, pears, and berries) and oats are rich in pectins, for example. Wheat, wheat bran, and other grains are high in cellulose.

Although not a nutrient (essential to life), fiber has many benefits. A diet high in fiber may lower cholesterol levels; reduce risk of colon cancer; help regulate blood sugar in diabetics; and prevent constipation, hemorrhoids, and diverticulosis (a sometimes precancerous condition in the colon) (15). Not all fibers provide the same preventive benefits. For example, pectin in apples and oats may help lower blood cholesterol, but doesn't appear to aid constipation. The fiber in whole grains does aid constipation, but doesn't affect blood cholesterol. For this reason, include several different fiber sources in the diet.

Did You Know That . . .

An ounce of kidney beans has 3 times more dietary fiber than an ounce of green beans. Raspberries have 4 times as much fiber as red cherries.

Fiber Sources

Good Fiber Sources	Poor Fiber Sources
whole wheat and whole grain breads	white bread, donuts, pastries, cake
whole wheat pastas	white flour pastas
brown rice	white rice
oatmeal and bran cereals	cream of wheat, cornflakes
dried beans	meat and eggs
dried peas and lentils	poultry and fish
fruit	fruit juices
vegetables	vegetable juices
potatoes	snack chips
nuts and seeds	butter, margarine, oils, sweeteners, jams, jellies, syrups

Functions and Sources of Some Dietary Fibers

Fiber Type	Functions	Sources
Cellulose and hemi-cellulose	Increase stool bulk Relieve constipation Prevent some digestive diseases May help prevent colon cancer	wheat bran whole grain cereals whole wheat bread
Pectin, guar gum, mucilages	Help normalize blood sugar May help lower blood cholesterol	apples, oats, legumes, peas, carrots, berries, pears

Source: Adapted from A. Chenault, *Nutrition and Health* (Holt, Rinehart and Winston, 1984), p. 49.

Good sources of fiber are whole grains, fruits and vegetables (including potatoes), legumes, nuts, and seeds. The refining process removes fiber, so whole wheat bread and brown rice are better choices than white bread and white rice; whole ground cornmeal is a better choice than refined, degermed cornmeal. Juices, which don't contain the fruit pulp, are poor sources, as are dairy products, meats, alcohol, fats, and sugars.

Americans currently consume about 11 grams of fiber daily, and it is recommended we consume 20 to 35 grams (16). This means many of us need to double or triple our intake of fiber. Following dietary guidelines to include daily 6 servings of grains, cereals, and legumes (choose whole grains and cereals) and 5 servings of fruits and vegetables will generally be adequate to meet the recommended intake for fiber.

GAME STRATEGY: CARBOHYDRATE

To meet current dietary recommendations, most of us need to double our intake of complex carbohydrates, increase fiber intake, and reduce our intake of refined sugar (17). The National Research Council recommends we obtain at least 55 percent of

(continued on p. 77)

The major sources of energy (calories) in the American diet are carbohydrates and fats. (Protein and alcohol also supply calories.) Carbohydrates are especially helpful in weight-reduction diets because, ounce for ounce, they contain about half as many calories as fats do.

Simple carbohydrates, such as sugars, and complex carbohydrates, such as starches, have about the same caloric content. But most foods high in sugar, such as candies and other sweets, contain little or no vitamins and minerals. On the other hand, foods high in starch, such as breads and other grain products, dry beans and peas, and potatoes, contain many of these essential nutrients.

Eat Foods with Adequate Starch and Fiber

Eating more foods containing complex carbohydrates can also help to add dietary fiber to your diet. The American diet is relatively low in fiber.

Dietary fiber is a term used to describe parts of plant foods which are generally not digestible by humans. There are several kinds of fiber with different chemical structures and biological effects. Because foods differ in the kinds of fiber they contain, it's best to include a variety of fiber-rich foods—whole-grain breads and cereals, fruits, and vegetables, for example.

Eating foods high in fiber has been found to reduce symptoms of chronic constipation, diverticular disease, and some types of "irritable bowel." It has been suggested that diets low in fiber may increase the risk of developing colon cancer. Whether this is true is not yet known.

How dietary fiber relates to cancer is one of many fiber topics under study. Some others are the fiber content of foods and the amount of fiber we need in our diets. Also being studied are whether fiber extracted from food has the same effect as that from intact food and the extent to which high fiber intakes may lead to trace mineral deficiency.

Advice for today: A diet containing whole-grain breads and cereals, fruits, and vegetables should provide an adequate intake of dietary fiber. Increase your fiber intake by eating more of these foods that contain fiber naturally, not by adding fiber to foods that do not contain it.

Source: U.S. Department of Agriculture Nutrition Information Services, *Home & Garden Bulletin*, No. 232, 1985.

FIGURE 3.4
Check Your Diet for Starch and Fiber

How Often Do You Eat:	Seldom or Never	1 or 2 Times a Week	3 to 4 Times a Week	Almost Daily
1. Several servings of breads, cereals, pasta or rice?	☐	☐	☐	☐
2. Starchy vegetables like potatoes, corn, peas, or dishes made with dry beans or peas?	☐	☐	☐	☐
3. Whole-grain breads or cereals?	☐	☐	☐	☐
4. Several servings of vegetables?	☐	☐	☐	☐
5. Whole fruit with skins and/or seeds (berries, apples, pears, etc.)?	☐	☐	☐	☐

The best answer for all of the above is ALMOST DAILY. Breads, cereals, and other grain products and starchy vegetables provide starch. Whole-grain products, fruits and vegetables, especially those with edible skins and seeds, are good sources of fiber.

Source: Adapted from U.S. Department of Agriculture *Home and Garden Bulletin* No. 232–4, April 1986.

FIGURE 3.5
Foods High in Fiber

To Obtain More Fiber . . .

Choose:	Instead of:
an orange	orange juice
whole wheat bread	enriched white bread
brown rice	white rice
bean burrito	beef taco
whole wheat spaghetti	white spaghetti
oatmeal	cream of wheat
lentil soup	chicken noodle soup
green peas	green beans
bran cereal	cornflakes
rye crackers	saltine crackers
an apple	apple juice
blackberries	grapes
baked potato	instant mashed potatoes

It takes this much white bread:

to get the same fiber in this much whole wheat bread:

It takes this much white rice:

to get the same fiber in this much brown rice:

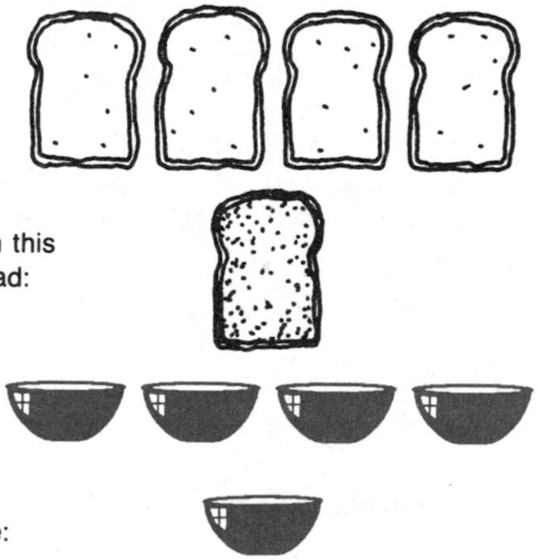

(Left) Most Americans need to increase their consumption of fiber. One relatively easy way to do this is to substitute higher fiber foods for some of those we ordinarily consume. (Right) Highly processed foods such as white bread and white rice contain substantially less fiber than their less-processed counterparts.

our calories from all carbohydrates combined (complex carbohydrates and sugar) (9).

To determine our own carbohydrate requirement, multiply our estimated daily calorie intake by 55 percent. This will tell us how many calories of carbohydrate we need. Then divide this number by 4 (4 calories are derived from every gram of carbohydrate). The number we now have is the number of grams of carbohydrate to include in our diet each day, more or less. Most of our carbohydrate should come from complex carbohydrates, not sugar. Use table 3.2 on page 60 to see which food group selections will meet your carbohydrate needs.

Nutrition experts exhibit less consensus on a recommended maximum level of sugar in the diet. How much sugar can be consumed before it becomes a problem? Certainly, one should be consuming foods to meet one's nutrient requirements on a regular basis before sugary foods are added in any great quantity. Following recent guidelines, this means 6 servings of breads, cereals, and legumes, 5 servings of fruits and vegetables, 2 servings of low-fat milk products, and 2 servings of protein foods daily (see table 2.3 on page 28 in chapter 2 for serving sizes).

The Dietary Guidelines for Americans simply state, "Avoid too much sugar" (14). Nutritional guidelines released in 1977 by a U.S. Senate Subcommittee on Diet and Health, as well as guidelines of several European countries, recommend sugar be kept to no more than 10 percent of calories, so that nutritious foods are not crowded out of the diet and likelihood of dental caries is lessened (18, 19). As an example, for someone consuming 2000 calories a day, 200 calories from sugar would be 10 percent (approximately 12.5 teaspoons of sugar), the amount in a small dessert plus a tablespoon of sugar, honey, or jam. A teaspoon of sugar or other sweetener contains 15 calories. By multiplying our estimated calorie intake by 10 percent, we can determine how many sugar calories to consume before we will exceed this 10 percent guideline. Use table 3.4 on page 71 to estimate how many teaspoons of sugar you currently consume, and how many sugar calories this provides in your diet. W

CHAPTER 4

Game Plan For A Healthy Diet

Protein • Fat

IN 1838 A DUTCH CHEMIST coined the word *protein*, meaning "that which takes first place," to describe these molecules essential to life. As one writer points out, although we think of DNA, the chemical of our genes, as the basis for our biological destiny, DNA functions solely to dictate what proteins are made and when in every living cell (1). It is the proteins themselves that are the constituents of tissues, hormones, antibodies, and the thousands of **enzymes** that regulate every reaction in the body, making life possible. In light of modern genetic research, the Dutch chemist's notion of protein proved quite apt.

PROTEIN

Proteins are large, complex, organic molecules consisting of linked chains of **amino acids**. A great variety of proteins exists because different amino acids combine in unique sequences to form individual proteins. For example, some are flexible and elastic like the protein of hair; others are firm and rigid like the protein of skin or fingernails because of the different sequences of amino acids. Twenty-two different amino acids are found in foods and all but nine of these are also made in the body. We must obtain these last nine **essential amino acids** from food.

Protein in the Body
Some of the protein we eat ends up in tissues such as muscle, as part of the structure. Additional protein is transformed into enzymes, the busy biological catalysts that speed up nearly every

Enzyme: A protein compound that facilitates biochemical reactions.

Amino acids: Nitrogen-containing compounds that are the building blocks of proteins. Twenty-two amino acids occur in proteins.

Essential amino acids: The 9 amino acids the body cannot form from other nitrogen-containing compounds and which must be obtained through the diet. They are phenylalanine, valine, threonine, tryptophan, isoleucine, methionine, histidine, leucine, and lysine.

78

Table 4.1 The Amino Acids: Building Blocks of Protein

Essential	Nonessential	
histidine	alanine	proline
isoleucine	arginine	serine
leucine	asparagine	tyrosine
lysine	aspartic acid	
methionine	cysteine	
phenylalanine	cystine	
threonine	glutamic acid	
tryptophan	glutamine	
valine	glycine	
	hydroxyproline	

The food we eat contains a total of 22 different amino acids, all but 9 of which are also manufactured in the body. These 9 "essential" amino acids must be obtained from our diet.

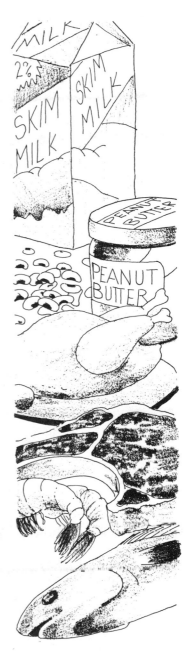

chemical reaction in the body. Protein is also used to make antibodies and hormones, to maintain a correct balance of fluids inside and outside cells, and to keep blood from becoming too acidic or too alkaline. Protein is used to build new tissue and to repair existing tissues on a daily basis. With all these crucial functions to carry out, thousands of different proteins are needed inside and outside every cell in the body.

Understandably, the misconception that large amounts of protein foods are needed for health is common. Although protein is a structural material in all cells, we need only 10 to 15 percent of our calories from protein. This is surprising when you consider that we cannot store excess protein eaten at a meal for more than a few hours.

Eating enough protein is necessary for health, but consuming protein in excess can have undesirable effects. Protein breakdown results in toxic nitrogen compounds that must be excreted from the body by way of the kidneys, so more water is needed when many protein foods are eaten (2). This is a particular concern for athletes, who need lots of fluids to replace their loss through sweat, and who may be eating 3 times the protein they need, mistakenly thinking this will help performance or muscle development. The result can be chronic underhydration that impairs both health and performance. Years of a high-protein diet

Table 4.2 A Day's Protein Need

3 ounces fish	21
2 cups skim milk	16
5 slices whole grain bread	15
	52 gm protein
1 cup navy beans	15
1 egg	6
1 oz cheddar cheese	7
2 cups skim milk	16
1 cup rice	4
5 slices whole grain bread	15
	63 gm protein

RDA for females: 44–50 grams
RDA for males: 59–63 grams

Source: U.S. Department of Agriculture, Handbook No. 456.

Eating enough protein is necessary for our health, but excessive amounts can have undesirable effects. The recommended daily allowance of protein for both males and females can be obtained from a relatively small amount of protein-rich foods such as those shown above.

contribute to excessive strain on the liver and kidneys and to loss of bone calcium (3). Animal protein foods are associated with increased risk for cancer and contribute to a high-fat intake (4).

Most Americans eat twice the protein they need (5). The RDA for adult women of average weight ranges from 44 to 50 grams a day and for adult men of average weight 59 to 63 grams. Recall that the National Research Council guidelines caution us not to overconsume protein foods to help prevent heart disease and cancer. Daily needs can be met with very few protein foods: 2 glasses of milk and 4 ounces of chicken supply enough for an average adult woman for a day; add a cup of baked beans and a slice of bread and enough protein is provided for a 170-pound man.

Protein in Foods

Protein-rich foods include fish, poultry, eggs, meat, milk products, and legumes. Vegetables and grains also provide small

(continued on p. 82)

Do professional athletes such as marathon runners, tennis players, and weight lifters need extra protein for peak performance? What about the person who exercises, the occasional athlete or even the "weekend warrior" (one who hits the pavement or the courts every Saturday or Sunday, only to return to a desk job on Monday)? Can extra protein enhance their athletic abilities?

Do Athletes and People Who Exercise Need Extra Protein?

While coaches have long insisted that loading up on protein is essential for maximum performance, nutritionists have insisted just as strongly that no healthy adult needs protein above the Recommended Dietary Allowance (RDA). However, newer information seems to show that neither belief is quite right. The fact is, *some* active people may need extra protein to stay in peak from, but for most, extra protein is a waste.

Energy for Exercise. It has been well established and accepted that *carbohydrates* are the major fuel the body uses during intense exercise. But since carbohydrate storage (in the liver and the muscles in the form of glycogen) is limited, it can be depleted rapidly—especially during exercise that occurs in intense, short sessions (like tennis, basketball or soccer).

Fat, on the other hand, is the major contributor to energy demands during low to moderately intense exercise and/or during prolonged exercise (longer than 60–90 minutes), when glycogen stores are likely to be depleted. This explains why jogging is so often recommended for getting rid of extra pounds—after a certain length of time, jogging burns fat.

So where does *protein* come in? Sports specialists in the past thought that protein had little to do with energy metabolism during exercise. But some recent findings indicate that protein may contribute more to the energy requirements of exercise than previously thought—as much as six to 15 percent of a person's energy needs, if the person begins exercise with low glycogen levels and/or exercises for more than one hour at a time.

So, those who exercise regularly for an hour or more each day require more than the RDA for protein. And, weight lifters do indeed require more than the RDA for protein—almost twice as much—to build their bulging biceps.

A Look at Protein Requirements. The RDA for all adults is .36 grams of protein per pound of body weight—that's about 47 grams of protein for an average woman, and 63 grams for an average man. The newest estimates of protein requirements for athletes range from .55 grams to .73 grams per pound of body weight. Endurance athletes such as long distance runners seem to require the least amount, while strength/power athletes such as weight lifters need the greatest.

Most Americans should *not* run out and buy protein powder—we already eat lots of protein. Sixteen-ounce steaks and double burgers with cheese are common dietary choices. A typical sirloin steak contains 69 grams of protein. A double burger with cheese has about 41 grams—almost a full day's requirement for a woman.

Indeed, government surveys indicate that we eat considerably more than the RDA of .36 grams per pound. We typically eat 44 to 75 percent above the RDA. This is plenty for even the most active athletes.

Don't Overload on Carbs. The only probable candidate for a protein deficit is one who tries to load up on carbohydrates at the expense of protein. No more than 55 to 70 percent of calories of an athlete's diet (or an active weekender's) should come from carbohydrates. The practice of carbohydrate loading, if done habitually, may indeed affect performance—in a negative way.

When such a large portion of the diet comes from carbohydrate, there is little room for extra protein. Probably at highest risk for less than optimum protein intake are strict vegetarians who exercise regularly. For them, protein supplements may be in order; they should seek the advice of a professional nutritionist.

As a general rule, 12 percent of calories as protein is enough for most people at the low end of the activity scale. For weight lifters and endurance athletes, about 18 percent of calories as protein should meet needs.

—Elizabeth Combier

Source: *Environmental Nutrition*, November 1987.

Vitamins: Organic (carbon-containing) compounds essential to life and needed in very small quantities. They are nutrients not made by the body and so must be obtained from food.

Trace minerals: Minerals in the body in very small quantities, each amounting to less than a total of 5 grams.

Incomplete protein: The protein, considered incomplete because it doesn't contain all 9 essential amino acids, that is found in legumes, grains, and vegetables.

amounts of protein and since these foods are generally eaten several times a day, they can contribute a considerable amount of protein to the diet. In addition to protein, these foods contribute many other nutrients. Meats and legumes in particular provide B **vitamins**, iron, zinc, and other **trace minerals**.

The protein in legumes, grains, and vegetables is termed **incomplete protein** because it does not contain all 9 essential amino acids. When eaten in combination with other protein foods in a balanced diet, however, these plant sources provide protein the body can use.

One of the important dietary recommendations of major health agencies and organizations is to reduce intake of fat to no more than 30 percent of calories. Because much of our current fat intake comes from protein-rich foods, choosing low-fat sources of protein can be important. Chicken and other poultry are only 20 to 30 percent fat whereas a T-bone steak and cheddar cheese have a whopping 75 to 80 percent fat content. Fish, which provides 10

**Table 4.3 Examples of Food Combinations
Providing Complete Protein**

Macaroni and Cheese	(Grain plus animal food)
Cereal and Milk	(Grain plus animal food)
Corn Tortilla and Beans	(Grain plus legume)
Tuna-Noodle Casserole	(Grain plus animal food)
Peanut Butter Sandwich	(Legume plus grain)
Rice and Black-eyed Peas	(Grain plus legume)
Rice Pudding	(Grain plus animal food)
Baked Beans and Brown Bread	(Legume plus grain)
Beans and Cheese	(Legume plus animal food)
Lentil Soup and Cornbread	(Legume plus grain)
Red Beans and Rice	(Legume plus grain)

The protein in legumes, grains, and vegetables is termed "incomplete" because it does not contain all 9 essential amino acids. When eaten in combination with other protein foods, however, these plant sources provide a complete protein diet.

percent of its calories as fat, is a wise choice as well. In addition, several types of fish contain fats called **omega-3 fatty acids** that may help protect against atherosclerosis and heart disease (6).

Protein for Vegetarians

For many, choosing a vegetarian diet is a preference based on ethical or religious reasons, since animal foods are not necessary for health. Even nonvegetarians are choosing to reduce their meat consumption in response to problems of world hunger, destruction of rain forest for cattle grazing, and the tremendous use of natural resources (water, fertilizer, grain crops) required to produce beef. It takes 2500 gallons of water and 16 pounds of edible food grains to produce 1 pound of beef, and 22 to 40 times the amount of fossil fuel as does grain to provide the same amount of protein (7).

There are solid health reasons for choosing to reduce intake of meat as well. Research shows that vegetarians have a lower incidence of chronic diseases such as cancer and heart disease, due in part to the lower fat, higher fiber, and higher fruit and vegetable content of the diet (8).

Omega-3 fatty acids:
Polyunsaturated fats found in fish oils and important in synthesis of hormonelike prostaglandins.

Table 4.4 Protein and Fat in Foods

	Percent of Calories from Protein	Percent of Calories from Fat
T-bone steak	20%	80%
Cheddar cheese	25%	75%
Peanut butter	17%	66%
Tuna packed in oil	34%	64%
Trimmed T-bone steak	50%	50%
Whole milk	21%	48%
Chicken	64%	31%
Fillet of sole	90%	10%
Skim milk	40%	Trace
Cooked dry beans	25%	Trace
Whole wheat bread	16%	Trace

Source: U.S. Department of Agriculture, Handbook No. 456.

Because much of our current fat intake comes from protein-rich foods, choosing low-fat sources of protein can be important. Foods such as fillet of sole, skim milk, and cooked dry beans are useful protein sources that contain very little fat.

Obtaining adequate protein on a vegetarian diet is not difficult if a few basic principles are followed. Animal foods (meat, poultry, fish, eggs, and milk products) supply all 9 essential amino acids, the protein building blocks needed by cells. Plant foods (vegetables, grains, legumes, nuts, and seeds) are missing or low in one or more amino acid. However, not all plant foods are missing or low in the same amino acids. By mixing and matching different plant foods together a person can take in all the essential amino acids. Two different foods that together provide a complete "set" of amino acids are termed **complementary protein** foods.

Traditional diets around the world include complementary protein foods. Corn tortillas eaten with beans are one example. Cornmeal is low in the amino acid lysine, but the beans provide this amino acid. The beans, on the other hand, are low in the amino acid methionine, which the cornmeal provides. Eaten together, these two incomplete protein foods provide a complete set of essential amino acids as usful to the body as those in a hamburger.

Complementary proteins: A term used to signify protein foods that together provide a complete set of essential amino acids, such as beans and a corn tortilla.

Small amounts of protein-rich animal foods such as milk, eggs, meat, or cheese eaten with plant foods also provide the complete spectrum of essential amino acids, thus meeting protein needs. This approach is common in Oriental diets, in which large amounts of incomplete protein foods such as rice and vegetables

(continued on p. 87)

Beans, Old or New, Win Fans Among Chefs and Nutritionists

Although people don't usually rhapsodize at cocktail parties about great bean dishes they have enjoyed lately, that is beginning to change. As new varieties of dried beans arrive on the market, and research unveils ever greater nutritional properties, beans are finding passionate advocates among culinarians.

When properly cooked, beans have a satisfying, sensual texture and tastes that range from buttery to tomatoey. Stylish restaurants are offering far more bean dishes than they did a few years ago, and the choices have expanded far beyond the basic white, black and red beans to varieties with variegated patterns and striking colors.

These discoveries have enhanced their already favorable status, but the nutritional benefits of beans have never been in doubt. In addition to providing a quarter of the body's daily protein requirements, with almost no fat, a cup of cooked beans has been found to help lower cholesterol. Indeed, the benefits of beans are equal to those of oats, which have lately received far more publicity for their cholesterol-lowering properties.

Dean & DeLuca, which supplies its own store in New York as well as other retailers and restaurants around the nation, has seen its bean sales triple in the last two years, said Philip Teverow, who buys all the items that carry the Dean & DeLuca label. Mr. Teverow declined to specify the amounts sold.

For the last few months, he has been stocking the store's shelves with old varieties of beans that are being rediscovered by growers. They have evocative names that reflect their coloring and unusual patterning—European soldier, Christmas lima, snowcap and appaloosa. Coming in the fall with be Jacob's cattle, painted lady and China yellow.

Most of the beans at Dean & DeLuca come from crops recently harvested in various parts of the United States. Although Mr. Teverow said that these beans do not need the customary soaking, which restores lost moisture, some cooks who have used them disagree.

The newly available beans may look unfamiliar, but they have similar nutritional advantages. And they probably will not offer any shocks to the palate. Mr. Teverow said beans of similar size and shape, regardless of coloration, tend to have the same taste and texture. The European soldier bean, for instance, which is white with a red marking that looks a bit like a soldier, tastes much like the red kidney bean, which is about the same size.

Although the more unusual beans may not offer brand-new tastes, Mr. Teverow says their novel appearance makes them popular and inspires people to add beans to their cooking repertory. "Color is as much a part of the development of a meal as the matching of the flavors," he said. All patterned beans lose some color in cooking, but most of them, except for tongues of fire and cranberry beans, retain their markings.

Others who specialize in resurrecting unusual, all-but-forgotten foods are also finding that beans are arousing a renewed interest. Georgeanne Brennan, a partner in Le Marché Seeds International, a supplier of unusual seeds in Dixon, Calif., said: "All of a sudden, people are really interested in them. I think they're really up-and-coming items."

Michael Romano, the chef at the Union Square

Cafe in New York, has put several bean dishes on his menu in the last few months, including a simple salad of white beans and a more complicated salad of beans and seafood. He says he believes that beans are appearing on more menus because they appeal to the current taste for hearty, bourgeois cooking.

Chez Panisse Cafe in Berkeley, Calif., has doubled its use of beans in the last five years, according to Catherine Brandel, a chef there. "I think people like them as an alternative to potatoes and noodles," she said.

At Zuni Cafe in San Francisco, the chef, Judy Rodgers, says she, too, is using more beans and finds that her customers like them. "I have 900 pounds of organic dried beans in my kitchen now," she said. "There isn't a place we don't use them, except in dessert."

After trying dried beans from recent crops, she said: "They have more taste. They're silky, as opposed to caky or pasty."

Both Zuni Cafe and Chez Panisse Cafe buy their beans from the Phipps Ranch in Pescadero, Calif., where Tommy and Valerie Phipps grow as many as 46 varieties, including old or "heirloom" beans like Jacob's cattle and yellow eye, and new varieties like the black scarlet runner. White cannellini beans are so popular with restaurants, Mr. Phipps said, that "we sold everything but the seed."

As retailers find more interest in beans, scientists are discovering more about their benefits. Since 1972, Dr. David J. A. Jenkins, a professor of medicine and nutritional science at the University of Toronto, has studied the effects of certain foods, including beans, on the development of diseases.

Dr. Jenkins has found that beans are as effective as oats in lowering cholesterol levels, but the decrease will vary from person to person. "We believe it is very difficult to make hard and fast rules," Dr. Jenkins said.

Dr. Jenkins has shown that many people can lower their cholesterol by 13 percent to 14 percent by eating two servings of beans each day. In his studies responses ranged from 7 percent to 27 percent, he said.

While certain foods lower cholesterol only because they contain insoluble fiber, beans have three characteristics that lower the lipid levels in the blood: their insoluble fiber and the composition of their protein and starch.

Dr. Jenkins noted that other "slow-release carbohydrate foods" lower blood lipids and also help control diabetes: lentils, split peas, oats, barley, dense-grain breads and pasta. "I'm not trying to knock the oats revolution," he said, "but just as one should have a mixed portfolio, one should have a varied diet."

Beans have other potent nutritional advantages. A cup of cooked navy beans, for example, has 15.8 grams of protein, or 26 percent of the amount an adult needs each day. That cup of beans also has a quarter of the iron needed daily, 63 percent of the folic acid and nearly 13 percent of the calcium.

Although beans contain amino acids, the components of proteins, they do not have sufficient amounts to make them a top-quality protein. For that reason, it is useful, although not necessary, to combine beans with grains. "Beans and rice make a good combination," said David Haytowitz, a nutritionist at the United States Department of Agriculture.

Indeed, nearly every culture has basic dishes in its cuisine that take advantage of that bean and grain combination, from the rice and beans of Mexico to the pasta and bean soups of Italy to the tofu and rice dishes of China.

Cookbooks that specialize in bean recipes often give tips for reducing intestinal gas, which makes many people reluctant to eat beans. But for every suggestion, there is an expert who believes that none of the recommendations work.

For his part, Dr. Jenkins, who has added beans to his diet since discovering their benefits, says he believes that the only way to avoid gas is to eat beans frequently. "It's something that tends in time to diminish," he said.

—*Trish Hall*

Source: *The New York Times*, January 25, 1989, p. C1.

Table 4.5 A Vegetarian Eating Plan for Adults

Food Group	Servings Daily	Serving Size
Whole grain breads and cereals	4–6	1 slice bread, 1 roll, 1 tortilla, $1/2$–$3/4$ cup cooked rice or pasta, 1 cup dry cereal
Protein-rich foods	2	1 cup legumes, 4 oz tofu, 2–3 oz meat analog, 2 eggs, 4 tbs peanut butter
Fruits and vegetables	5 (include 1 cup dark greens for iron and one or more servings rich in vitamin C)	1 medium piece fruit, $1/2$ cup juice, $1/2$ cup cooked vegetable or fruit, 1 cup raw vegetable
Milk products	2–3	1 cup skim or low fat milk, yogurt, or soy milk fortified with vitamin B12, $1^{1}/2$ oz cheese

Unlike animal foods, no single plant food contains all nine of the essential amino acids. However, obtaining adequate protein on a vegetarian diet is not difficult if one mixes and matches different plant foods in combinations that together supply all nine of these essential nutrients.

are combined with small amounts of meat or fish in a variety of dishes. The result is a diet low in fat but adequate in protein.

Foods that eaten together provide all the essential amino acid building blocks of protein include:

1. Grains with legumes. Examples are bread and peanut butter, a tortilla with beans.

2. Nuts with legumes. Examples are a sandwich spread made with sunflower seeds and lentils and a Middle Eastern falafel sandwich with sesame seed tahini sauce (a spicy, fried, garbanzo bean mixture served in pita bread).

3. Small amounts of milk, cheese, or meat with larger amounts of grains or legumes. Examples are macaroni and cheese, cereal with milk, tuna noodle casserole, refried beans with cheese, and Oriental rice dishes containing vegetables and meat, chicken, or seafood.

FATS

Fat—essential nutrient or maligned substance? The answer is both. It makes up a suprisingly large portion of the typical American diet—37 percent of the calories on average. Fats, or lipids, are organic compounds consisting of hydrogen, carbon, and oxygen and are found in both animal and plant foods. Fats in foods exist primarily in the form of compounds called **triglycerides**. Cholesterol is not technically a fat but a fat-like substance in animal foods. The body can manufacture both triglycerides and cholesterol to meet most of its needs from other food components, so both these compounds will be found in blood and body tissues even if the diet is low in them.

Because it has numerous essential functions, fat or triglycerides should supply at least 10 percent of our calories. However, because fat is found in many foods and tastes so good, most of us take in much more.

As mentioned earlier, it is recommended that fat be limited to 30 percent of calories to lower risk for cardiovascular disease and

(continued on p. 94)

FIGURE 4.1
Fat Consumption

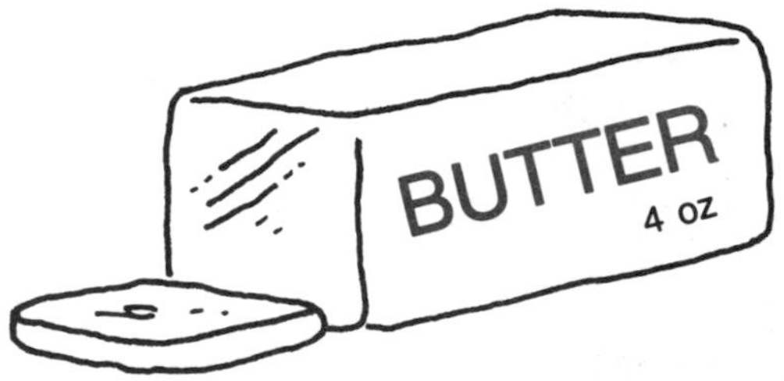

Triglyceride: A fat compound found in foods and made in the body, consisting of a carbon "backbone" to which are attached three fatty acids.

The average American fat intake: 24 teaspoons a day—equivalent to a stick of butter.

Lessons We Can Learn From Vegetarians

It wasn't all that long ago that the word *vegetarian* conjured up an image of a stringy-haired flower child in a gauze shirt munching happily on raw sesame seeds or some equally unlikely health food. But not any more. Vegetarianism has gone mainstream. A new proliferation of vegetarian restaurants, convenience foods, and cookbooks now offer meatless meals that entice rather than turn off. Seaweed, tofu, and soyburgers have given way to appetizing dishes like hearty eggplant parmigiana and raucous New Orleans-style red beans and rice.

None of this, of course, is tangible proof that the United States is soon to convert wholesale to vegetarianism. But for some people the focus is shifting away from meat as the centerpiece of meals. And that trend away from animal foods and toward plant foods (consumption of fresh vegetables is up 30 percent since 1970 according to the Department of Agriculture) has plenty to recommend it. Why? As a group, those who fill their plates with fruits, vegetables, and grains rather than with large amounts of foods that come from animals are at a much lower risk for the most common "American" illnesses: heart disease, colon cancer, diabetes, hypertension, and obesity.

What makes such a diet so salubrious? Is it hard to follow? Is it necessary to shun meat, poultry, and fish to enjoy good health, or can a happy compromise be made? We think the answers are more palatable than you may imagine.

The benefits of vegetables

One of the biggest pluses of an eating plan in which plant foods are the mainstay is its low fat content. Indeed, both the American Heart Association and the American Cancer Society have issued messages that emphasize low-fat, high-carbohydrate foods, such as fruits and vegetables, and deemphasize animal foods, which are comparatively high in fat.

Fortunately, it is not necessary to go completely vegetarian to enjoy the benefits afforded by a vegetarian regimen. Just changing the proportions of foods from animal and plant sources will help keep fat out of your diet—and your arteries. A traditional 10-ounce sirloin steak intended for one person, for example, could easily be turned into a 5-ounce serving for each of two people.

The "hole" that's left on the plate can be filled with, say, a heftier salad, a larger serving of broccoli or spinach, or even a second baked potato or a second corn on the cob. As long as that extra potato or corn is not "dressed" with more than a teaspoon or two of margarine, the savings in fat calories will remain substantial. Indeed, cutting out 5 ounces of steak results in eating up to 120 fewer calories as fat. Adding two teaspoons of margarine to a potato or a corn on the cob, both of which are fat-free, will put back only 70 calories of fat—most of it unsaturated, unlike the fat in the beef, which is saturated. Moreover, substituting a potato or corn or any other vegetable, fruit, or grain for some portion of beef, poultry, or fish will usually result in big money savings as well.

Don't be concerned that by cutting down on animal foods you may be risking deficiencies in many of the nutrients they contain. It is that concern, by the way, that leads many animal flesh eaters to envision vegetarians as anemic specimens barely able to keep pace with those around them.

But most vegetarians do not have any more nutritional problems than the rest of the population. It is true that meat, poultry, and fish are excellent sources of protein and iron as well as the B vitamins and several other nutrients. But legumes and grains, in the right combinations, can provide enough protein. And dried beans and dried fruits, such as raisins, contribute small amounts of iron. Whole-grain products also supply iron as well as B vitamins and other minerals.

Then, too, cutting back on flesh foods does not mean giving up other animal-derived foods such as eggs and low-fat dairy products, both of which supply high-quality protein along with a host of other essential nutrients. In fact, 90 percent of the 6 to 8 million Americans who call themselves vegetarians do eat eggs as well as cheese and drink milk (they are technically known as lacto-ovo vegetarians). Certainly, if these vegetarians can meet their nutritional needs, people who continue to eat meat but in smaller portions should have no problems.

Of course, meeting nutritional requirements does not address the fact that a piece of meat or poultry the size of a deck of cards rather than the size of *TV Guide*—the size many Americans are accustomed to—may appear paltry, even if the rest of the plate is loaded with more vegetables. Fortunately, there's an easy way around that problem: Instead of preparing meat or poultry as the main dish, make more use of recipes in which it is sliced, cubed, or chopped and combined with pasta or rice—as is often done in various ethnic cuisines. That kind of preparation "stretches" a smaller amount of animal food across the plate and creates a heartier look than you'd get from a reduced-size serving of beef or chicken occupying the spot that larger portions have always filled.

Creating ethnic cuisine, incidentally, which tends to use flesh foods as a condiment rather than as the centerpiece of a meal, does not require any more than the most rudimentary cooking skills. A Chinese stir fry, for example, can be made simply by slicing a few ounces of beef or chicken breast into thin strips, sautéeing with chopped pepper, mushrooms, and water chest-nuts, and serving over rice. Meat sauce for Italian pasta—for which almost everyone has a recipe—is another logical choice for "stretching" meat; each person eating a plate of spaghetti topped with meat sauce will end up with much less ground beef than if he or she ate a hamburger or a generous slice or two of meatloaf. And if you brown the beef and drain the fat before adding it to the sauce, the meal will be even lower in fat.

Proof that the changes pay off

Is it really worthwhile to alter lifelong eating habits and adopt the view that steak and other meats do not need to fill up a third of the plate for a meal to be nutritious and satisfying? That is, can the new approach really make a difference?

The answer to that is an unequivocal "yes."

Some of the strongest evidence that a diet rich in plant foods and sparing of animal foods confers a variety of health benefits comes from observations of Seventh Day Adventists, many of whom eat no animal flesh. Compared to those who eat the typical high-fat American diet, members of this religious sect have a dramatically lower rate of heart disease than Americans as a whole.

Indeed, one group of researchers in California found that the death rate from coronary disease in male members of the sect is as low as half that in the average California male. Undoubtedly, the fact that Seventh Day Adventists are non-smokers also contributes to the low death rate, since smoking, high blood pressure, and high blood cholesterol are three major risk factors for heart disease. But diet apparently plays an integral role, since the rate of heart disease among Seventh Day Adventists who are not vegetarians was found to be three times higher than that for their vegetarian counterparts.

The low-fat vegetarian diet of many Seventh Day Adventists may also be what makes them half as likely as other Americans to develop colon and rectal cancer. Their rate of cancer of the breast, prostate, pancreas, and ovaries is much smaller too. But less fat is probably just part of the equation. Diets that favor large portions of fruits, vegetables, and grains are also beneficial to health because they are low in dietary cholesterol and high in fiber. The *soluble* fiber found in oats, fruits, and vegetables, including legumes, can lower high levels of cholesterol in the blood. And the *insoluble* fiber in whole grains like wheat, besides preventing constipation, may be protective against some tumors (although the jury is still out on that one).

A high-fiber diet can also help people who have diabetes control their blood sugar. For years the American Diabetes Association has encouraged diabetics to adhere to a diet that includes plenty of vegetables, whole grains, and fruit—high-fiber foods that are rich in complex carbohydrates—to help keep their blood sugar "on an even keel."

Along with fiber, fruits and vegetables contain

beta-carotene and indoles, both of which may be of some value on their own in preventing cancer. In fact, a large body of research on animals and humans suggests that beta-carotene, a vitamin-A-like compound found in deep orange and deep green fruits and vegetables such as apricots, sweet potatoes, cantaloupe, broccoli, and spinach, may be helpful in warding off a few types of cancer. And preliminary studies indicate that potentially cancer-fighting indoles, present in cruciferous vegetables like cauliflower and Brussels sprouts, may inhibit the growth of some cancers as well.

Aside from their possible protection against cancer, plant foods have the distinction of supplying a rich array of vitamins and minerals needed in the diet without providing a lot of calories. Perhaps that's why vegetarians are more likely than other Americans to be slender, which in itself affords protection against high blood pressure, heart disease, and diabetes. Indeed, strict vegetarians often weigh as much as 20 pounds less than their nonvegetarian counterparts. In a nation where obesity is a major, if not *the* major, nutritional problem—32 million Americans are more than 20 percent above the weight deemed "ideal" for their height and frame size—that's a statistic worth keeping in mind.

Tips for staying in the pink

The strictest vegetarians—a small minority called vegans who abstain from eating not only the flesh of animals but also dairy products and eggs—need to pay closer attention than others to their intake of certain nutrients in order to avoid deficiencies. Indeed, while no one can argue against the advantages of limiting the amount of fat in the diet, including the fat in meat and certain dairy products, those who follow strict vegetarian diets may very well be at increased risk for a variety of nutritional problems that meat and dairy eaters do not have to worry about.

That's not to say it's impossible to put together a reasonably well balanced vegan diet If you have a particularly good grasp of the science of nutrition. But diets that do not include any animal foods whatsoever often lack calories along with essential vitamins and minerals and are usually inadequate for growing children along with anyone else with special nutritional needs.

Lacto-ovo vegetarians and semi-vegetarians (the people who are cutting down on flesh foods) do not have to be as concerned as vegans about meeting nutritional requirements, but an understanding of the needs of strict vegetarians will help them avoid any potential problems in their own no-meat or low-meat diets.

One nutrient vegans must consider more carefully than others is calcium because the dairy products they eschew are the best sources. Vegans, or anyone else looking for that mineral, will find some of it in broccoli. One large stalk of broccoli provides more than 10 percent of the recommended adult allowance. Collard greens and mustard greens supply appreciable levels, too, but those two vegetables are hard to come by. Small amounts of calcium can be found in the likes of dried beans, oranges, cabbage, and pumpkin. Unfortunately, the calcium in plant foods may not be absorbed as readily as the calcium in animal foods. That's why it's important for vegans to eat generous portions of calcium-containing vegetables.

As for iron, it too is found in a wide variety of plant foods, including legumes. A cup of dried beans, peas, or lentils contains about 5 milligrams of iron, or just under a third of the RDA of 18 milligrams for women and half of the RDA of 10 milligrams for men. But similar to calcium, the iron in plant foods is not well absorbed, something to consider in light of the fact that even meat eaters lack iron in their diets.

To improve iron absorption, a strict vegetarian, or anyone else, can eat a food containing vitamin C at the same time as a food that contains iron. Putting vitamin-C rich tomato sauce over pasta fortified with iron, for instance, allows the body to utilize more of the iron available. Abstaining from tea and coffee when eating foods that supply iron will help, too, since both beverages contain substances that inhibit the body's absorption of iron.

Vegans also need to be aware that the protein in plant foods, as opposed to the protein in animal foods such as beef, milk, cheese, and eggs, is not "complete." That is, one or another plant food by itself cannot provide the body with all the compounds that make up the proteins humans require for building and maintaining body tissues. Fortunately, the "incomplete" proteins found in plants can be combined for "completeness." Putting together red beans with rice, for instance, turns two sources of incomplete protein into one complete source. Split pea soup and a crusty slice of rye bread—another legume-grain combination—makes for another "full" complement.

In addition to a planning strategy for protein, vegetarians have to pay particular attention to their intake of vitamin B_{12} because that nutrient, without which pernicious anemia develops, is naturally available in animal foods only. One way to insure that the need for vitamin B_{12} is met is to eat cereals fortified with it. Many soy milk products are also fortified with vitamin B_{12}. Fortification or not, however, vegetarians who go without eggs and dairy products would do well to consult a knowledgeable physician about taking vitamin B_{12} supplements, or a multivitamin mineral supplement that contains that nutrient, since B_{12} in fortified cereals and soy foods is often not provided in large enough amounts.

That same doctor's visit should also include a discussion about whether supplements of vitamin D are necessary. People who do not drink milk may be at risk of a vitamin D deficiency, since it is just about the only food fortified with that nutrient. It's true that exposure to the sun allows the body to synthesize vitamin D, but not everyone, especially those living in northern climates, gets the amount of sunlight necessary to make all the vitamin D the body needs.

Vegetarian for a day

The one-day menu below shows how a nutrition-conscious lacto-ovo vegetarian might plan his meals. Of the 1,800 calories provided, less than 30 percent come from fat, which is in keeping with the recommendation of the American Heart Association and The National Cholesterol Education Program. In addition, these dishes contribute fewer than 300 milligrams of cholesterol, all the essential vitamins and minerals, including iron and calcium, and more than 20 grams of fiber.

The American Cancer Institute says we should take in at least that much fiber every day.

Breakfast
1 cup bran cereal
1 cup lowfat (1%) milk
1 slice whole-wheat toast with 1 tsp tub margarine
1/2 grapefruit
coffee or tea

Lunch
1 cup split pea soup made with lowfat (1%) milk
1 slice rye bread with 1 tsp tub margarine
Spinach salad
  1 cup chopped raw spinach
  1/2 tomato
  1/4 cup shredded carrot
  1/2 chopped hard-boiled egg
  2 tbsp walnuts
  1 tbsp raisins
  1 tbsp low-cal dressing of choice

Midafternoon snack
1 banana

Dinner
Low-fat pasta primavera
  1 cup pasta mixed with 1/4 cup each broccoli flowerets, sliced mushrooms, and sliced zucchini
  1/3 cup kidney beans
  Chill and top with 1 tbsp Parmesan cheese and 2 tbsp low-cal Italian dressing
1 slice whole-grain bread with 1 tsp tub margarine
1 cup low-fat (1%) milk
1 cup strawberries

Snack
3 gingersnaps
1 cup low-fat (1.5%) vanilla yogurt mixed with 1/2 cup fresh blueberries

Besides paying close attention to vitamins B_{12} and D along with calcium, iron, and protein, vegans as well as lacto-ovo vegetarians and semi-vegetarians would do well to follow a few steps that will insure better nutrition all around:

• When cooking with water, always keep the amount to a minimum (steam rather than boil if possible) to prevent nutrients from leaching out. Even iron can be lost from a vegetable submerged in boiling water.

- Try to keep the skins of vegetables and fruits on. But if you must remove them, peel as thinly as possible. Many vitamins (and much of the flavor) are directly under the skin.
- Use high-fat dairy products such as cream, whole milk, and hard cheese sparingly. Limiting the amount of flesh foods you eat will not remove enough fat to eliminate the need to pay attention to the fat content of other items. Indeed, butter is just about 100 percent fat. Cheeses are often 70 percent fat or more. And fat contributes 50 percent of the calories in whole milk. Better choices are low-fat or nonfat yogurt, skim milk, low-fat cottage cheese, reduced-fat hard cheeses, and part-skim semisoft cheeses.

A word about vegetarian cookbooks

People who are somewhat at a loss as to how to reduce the amount of meat in meals—or to get flesh foods out of some dinner dishes altogether—may want to add a vegetarian cookbook to their collection. But how do you choose the right one? Indeed, vegetarian cookbooks now take up nearly as much space in bookstores as diet cookbooks.

Unfortunately, many books devoted to vegetarian cuisine do not offer recipes that are any more healthful than those in other cookbooks—despite the wholesome-looking, grainy texture of the pages, the fanciful script, and the earth tones many of them use to denote that their menus are "pure" or "natural" or "go back to basics." In fact, some recommend butter over margarine, cream or whole milk over low-fat or skim, inordinate amounts of high-fat cheeses, and more egg yolks than most people normally use.

A recipe for fettuccine Alfredo in Anna Thomas's The Vegetarian Epicure: Book Two (Alfred A. Knopf: New York, 1978; softcover, $10.95), for instance, calls for 1½ cups of heavy cream, 1½ cups of grated parmesan cheese, ½ cup of butter, and 2 egg yolks. Since it is meant to serve six, that amounts to 235 milligrams of dietary cholesterol per person (close to the daily limit recommended by the American Heart Association) and 418 calories from fat alone—much of

it of the saturated variety that is prone to clog arteries.

That's not to say that the fettuccine Alfredo in Thomas's book contains more fat and cholesterol than a recipe in any nonvegetarian cookbook or is not delicious. After all, fat is indigenous to the dish. Nor does it take away from the many other dishes in her work that are low in fat as well as healthful overall (the roasted eggplant and peppers in oil, for instance). It's simply a caution that just because a recipe appears in a vegetarian cookbook, it is not automatically healthful.

So consider the ingredients in recipes carefully. Decide whether you can substitute egg whites for yolks, milk for cream, and part-skim for whole-milk cheeses. If you cannot do that for at least some of the items without destroying the taste of the dish, you may want to move on to one that's low in cream, eggs, and cheeses to begin with.

With those suggestions in mind, you're safe making use of just about any vegetarian cookbook, including The Vegetarian Epicure, which contains 325 recipes for everything from bread and muffins to Indian, Italian, and Mexican cuisine. Recipes closer to home can be found in American Harvest: Regional Recipes for the Vegetarian Kitchen, by Nava Atlas (Fawcett Columbine: New York, 1987; softcover, $9.95). That book will take you from a southern version of potatoes with collard greens (no salt pork or bacon needed) to "Texas Caviar," a marinated black-eyed pea salad.

Those looking for gourmet vegetarian recipes should look to The Greens Cook Book, by Deborah Madison with Edward Espe Brown (Bantam Books: New York, 1987; hardcover, $19.95). Straight from the kitchen of San Francisco's popular vegetarian restaurant, Greens, come recipes for such delights as jicama-orange salad and cannelloni with greens and walnut sauce.

One of the best bets with a view to good nutrition, however, is The New Laurel's Kitchen (Ten Speed Press: Berkeley, California, 1986; softcover, $15.95), by Laurel Robertson, Carol Flinders, and Brian Ruppenthal. The back of this 500-recipe book gives the calories, amount of fat, protein, carbohydrate, calcium, iron, sodium, and other minerals and vitamins for every dish listed. Along with the recipes are sections on Controlling Your Weight, Nutrition in Later Years, Diet Against Disease, Conserving Nutrients in the Kitchen, and discussions about which foods contain which nutrients and why they are needed.

The recipes themselves range from hearty carrot soup made with milk and vegetable stock (rather than cream) to the more exotic Nori Maki Sushi, a Japanese dish with no less than 10 different vegetables, including lightly steamed asparagus, bell peppers, and spinach. Also included in the cadre of vegetarian delicacies are green bean stroganoff, parsley stuffed potatoes (prepared with yogurt instead of sour cream, which has much more fat), and Brussels Sprout-Squash Casserole.

Source: *Tufts University Diet and Nutrition Letter,* Vol. 6, No. 5, July 1988.

Did You Know That . . .

If you chill soups and stews after cooking, you can skim off the fat that congeals on the top, and eat healthier.

Prostaglandins: Hormonelike compounds synthesized in the body from fatty acids with roles in numerous body processes.

cancer. All the cholesterol needed by the body can be made by the liver and we do not need to take in any through the diet. Because excessive dietary cholesterol plays a role in heart disease, experts recommend no more than 300 milligrams be consumed daily.

Fat in the diet does not necessarily become fat in the body. Remember that excess calories from any source (protein, carbohydrate, alcohol, or fat) can be stored as fat tissue. But gram for gram, fat does contain more than twice the calories of protein or carbohydrate, and a diet high in fat is likely to be high in calories. A gram of fat contains 9 calories (and new research shows some fats contain 11 calories per gram!), compared to only 4 calories in a gram of protein or carbohydrate. A teaspoon of sugar yields only 15 calories, whereas a teaspoon of fat yields about 40 calories. Three ounces of sirloin steak contain 406 calories, 64 calories provided by protein and 242 calories provided by fat.

Functions of Fats

In spite of concern about heart disease and cancer from overconsumption, fats and cholesterol are essential to life. Fats are used to make hormones (for example, the male and female sex hormones estrogen, progesterone, and testosterone), cell membranes and nerves; to cushion organs; and to provide an immediate and a reserve fuel source. Certain fats are made into hormone-like compounds called **prostaglandins** which regulate several processes, including the deposit of fat in blood vessels. Fats in food also help the fat-soluble vitamins A, D, E, and K pass from the digestive tract into the blood. A small amount of fat at each meal provides satiety, or the feeling our food is staying with us (which indeed it is, since fat slows down digestion).

Cholesterol is needed to manufacture sex hormones and is an essential component of brain and nerve cells. It is also a component of the fat deposits that can form in arteries over time and contribute to cardiovascular disease.

Table 4.6 The Percent of Fat Calories in Food

More than 90% fat	Bacon, mayonnaise, margarine, butter, cooking and salad oils, lard, cream, vegetable shortening, baking chocolate, olives
80–90% fat	Salad dressings, cream cheese, nuts, avocados, coconut, corned beef, sausages
50–80% fat	Beef, lamb, pork, veal, canadian bacon, ham, frankfurters, cheese (American, Swiss, cheddar, jack, etc.), peanut butter, ice cream, potato chips, chocolate candy, tuna in oil
35–50% fat	Round steak, lean ground beef, whole milk, fried chicken and fish, most cookies, crackers, cakes, donuts
20–35% fat	Low-fat milk and yogurt, liver, pancakes, muffins
Less than 20% fat	Skim milk, buttermilk, frozen yogurt, chicken without skin, broiled fish, seafood (shrimp, scallops), tuna in water, beans, peas, lentils, bread, breakfast cereals (except granola), grains, rice, pasta, fruits, vegetables (except avocados and olives)

The current guideline for fat intake is not more than 30 percent of the day's total calories. Balance high-fat foods with larger quantities of low-fat foods.

Chemistry of Fats

Most dietary fats are chemical triglycerides whether they are solid, like lard, or liquid, like corn oil. A triglyceride is a carbon backbone with three **fatty acids** attached. Triglycerides in food are called saturated or unsaturated depending on the type of fatty acids that predominate. For example, a saturated fat contains triglycerides with hydrogen atoms filling all available spots on the chemical chain of the fatty acid. An unsaturated fat contains triglycerides with one or more empty spots on the chemical chain of the fatty acid. Unsaturated fats are either **polyunsaturated** (many empty spots on the chain) or **monounsaturated** (one empty spot on the chain).

In general, saturated fats are found in animal foods, and unsaturated fats in plant foods. Corn and safflower oils are polyunsaturated, as are most plant oils. Exceptions are olive oil,

Fatty acid: Chemical compounds containing carbon, hydrogen, and oxygen. They form part of the triglycerides in food and in the body and can be saturated, polyunsaturated, or monounsaturated.

Polyunsaturated fat: A type of triglyceride rich in polyunsaturated fatty acids such as linoleic and linolenic acid that contains several points of unsaturation in its chemical structure. Safflower, soy, corn, sesame, cottonseed, and sunflower oils are rich in polyunsaturated fatty acids.

Monounsaturated fat: A type of triglyceride, rich in monounsaturated fatty acids such as oleic acid, that contains only one point of unsaturation in its chemical structure. Olive, peanut, and canola oils are rich in monounsaturated fats.

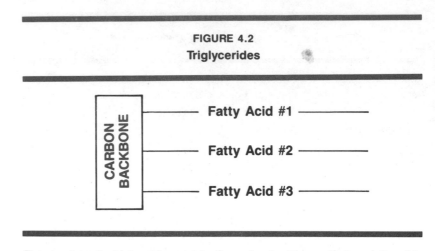

FIGURE 4.2
Triglycerides

The structure of a triglyceride consists of a carbon backbone with three fatty acids attached. The carbon backbone is a compound called glycerol, hence the term, "tri glycer ide."

peanut oil, and canola or rapeseed oil, which are primarily monounsaturated oils. The fats in beef, pork, lamb, and milk products contain a high percentage of saturated fatty acids, as do the tropical oils, palm and coconut. The labels on many processed foods list these latter two fats as ingredients. Several major food companies have now begun to phase out use of these oils in baked products because of consumer interest in eating fewer saturated fats.

With modern food technology, unsaturated oils are often turned into harder, more saturated fats by pumping hydrogen through them to fill up the empty spots on the fatty acid chains. This process is called **hydrogenation**, and results in a more saturated fat. Corn oil is hydrogenated to make it into margarine. The oil becomes solid rather than liquid at room temperature, and more spreadable (who wants to drizzle oil on their toast?) Margarines that come in tubs rather than sticks are less saturated and therefore more liquid at room temperature. They are a better choice for people interested in reducing saturated fat intake.

Fats in Foods

Hydrogenation: A process of adding hydrogen to unsaturated fatty acids to make them more saturated and solid.

Foods high in fat include beef, lamb, pork, butter, margarine, oils, cream, whole milk, cheese, ice cream, fried foods, nuts, avocados, snack chips, crackers, cookies, pastries, and many desserts. Cholesterol occurs only in animal foods. Foods high in cholesterol

FIGURE 4.3
Fatty Acids

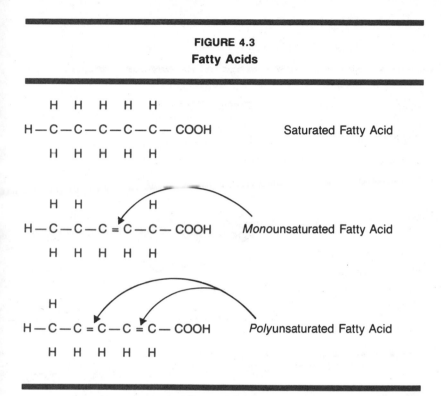

The structure of a fatty acid depends on the chemical bonding of its carbon component and the absence of hydrogen atoms in the chemical chain. A fatty acid with one double bond is monounsaturated, and with two or more double bonds is polyunsaturated. These double bonds take the place of hydrogen atoms.

include organ meats such as liver, shellfish, whole milk, meats, and poultry.

Much of the fat and cholesterol in the American diet comes from meat (9). Although meat is an excellent source of protein and other nutrients, most meats contain more fat than protein. One's protein need can be supplied by 2 to 3 ounces of meat at a meal, but 2 or 3 times that amount is commonly consumed. A 3-ounce hamburger provides 235 calories, 82 calories from protein and 153 calories from fat, and 231 milligrams of cholesterol.

The fat in meats, poultry, fish, eggs, milk products, and packaged, processed foods is often hidden it is not visible in the way that butter, gravy, and the whipped cream on a hot fudge sundae are and one may not realize how much fat is really there. A piece of cheddar cheese does not look "fatty," but contains 2 teaspoons per ounce. An avocado contains over 7 teaspoons of fat.

(continued on p. 99)

Table 4.7 Dietary Fat & Fatty Acid Proportions

Key:

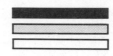

Saturated Fatty Acids
Monounsaturated Fatty Acids
Polyunsaturated Fatty Acids

Fats with large amounts of saturated fatty acids include:

Coconut oil

Palm kernel oil

Dairy fats
  butter, cream, cheese, milk

Palm oil

Meat fat
  beef fat, pork fat, lard

Poultry fat
  chicken fat, turkey fat

Fats with large amounts of monounsaturated fatty acids include:

Olive oil

Peanut oil

Hydrogenated vege-
  table shortening

Margarine, stick

Fats with large amounts of polyunsaturated fatty acids include:

Margarine, soft
  liquid vegetable oil as the first
  ingredient

Cottonseed oil

Soybean oil

Corn oil

Sunflower oil

Safflower oil

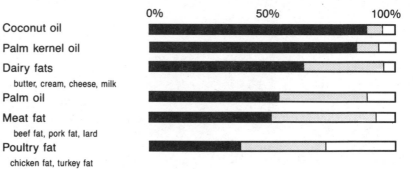

Note: All fats, whether they contain mainly saturated fatty acids, monounsaturated fatty acids, or polyunsaturated fatty acids, provide the same number of calories: 9 calories per gram.

Source: U.S. Department of Agriculture, Nutrition and Information Services, *Home and Garden Bulletin,* No. 232–8.

Table 4.8 Fat Consumption

If Total Calories Are:	Eat No More Than This Many Grams or Teaspoons of Fat
1200	40 grams or 8 teaspoons
1500	50 grams or 10 teaspoons
1800	60 grams or 12 teaspoons
2100	70 grams or 14 teaspoons
2400	80 grams or 16 teaspoons
2700	90 grams or 18 teaspoons

We are advised to eat no more than 30 percent of our daily calories as fat. Here's how that guideline translates into grams and teaspoons of fat.

The proliferation of fast-food restaurants and processed foods in the supermarket has also added to our fat consumption. Foods that start out low in fat can wind up very high in fat after being processed into another form. For example, a large baked potato contains approximately 160 calories and virtually no fat. Eaten as french fries, the calories increase to 620, 45 percent provided by fat. Eaten as potato chips, the calories increase to 1288, 63 percent of which come from fat!

The Bad News About Fat

The relationship of dietary fat to atherosclerosis (the accumulation of fatty deposits in blood vessels) and cardiovascular disease is an area of continuing research. When deposits of fatty substances build up in blood vessels, circulation of blood with its vital load of oxygen is impaired. Atherosclerosis can result in poor circulation and death by heart attack or stroke if the heart or brain are deprived of oxygen by their fat-clogged blood vessels. Diseases of the heart and blood vessels are the cause of half of all deaths in industrialized countries (10).

Many factors are involved in development of heart disease, including smoking, heredity, overweight, hypertension, lack of exercise, and diet. A high intake of saturated fat, not cholesterol, is considered the biggest dietary contributor to atherosclerosis (11). When many saturated fats are present, the liver manufactures more of the compounds (**lipoproteins**) that move cholesterol throughout the body. With more saturated fats in the diet, the blood levels of cholesterol increase and fatty plaques can wind up on blood vessel walls.

Lipoproteins: A compound of protein and lipids manufactured by the liver which moves cholesterol throughout the body.

Table 4.9 Types of Fat Found in Various Food Sources

Types of Fat	Food Sources
Cholesterol found in foods of animal origin	egg yolk, meat, fish, poultry, and milk and milk products

Saturated fatty acids
  found in largest proportions in
  fats of animal origin, but also in
  plants
	meat, poultry, whole milk, cream, butter, cheese, and coconut and palm oils

Monounsaturated fatty acids
  found in both animals and
  plants
	olive and peanut oil, and hydrogenated vegetable shortenings and margarines

Polyunsaturated fatty acids
  found in largest proportions in
  fats of plant origin
	sunflower, corn, soybean, safflower, and cottonseed oils, and some kinds of fish

Source: *The Dietary Guidelines: Seven Ways to Help Yourself to Good Health and Good Nutrition,* The American Dietetic Association, 1987.

Different types of food contain different types of fats. Cholesterol is found only in foods of animal origin. The same is generally true of saturated fatty acids (with the notable exception of the tropical oils). Polyunsaturated fatty acids are most common among fats of plant origin while monounsaturated fatty acids are found in both animals and plants.

The precise impact of dietary fat and cholesterol on the risk of heart disease remains a subject of debate among health experts, although most major health agencies believe the impact is clearly significant enough to warrant advising the general public to reduce fat and cholesterol intake. Some experts follow the medical model and argue that only those who have high blood cholesterol or who are at high risk for developing heart disease should be told to lower their fat intake. Other experts, following the public health model, counter that since over 50 percent of the population has blood cholesterol above desireable levels and half of all deaths are due to heart disease, it is prudent to advise everyone to consume a low-fat, low-cholesterol diet. It does no harm, may do a lot of good, and is advised for cancer prevention anyway. In addition, by the time elevated blood cholesterol is detected, damage to the arteries may have already occurred. The National Research Council states, "A large and convincing body

(continued on p. 103)

Cholesterol: Is It Worth the Bother?

If you're over 50, should you worry about cholesterol? If you're a woman, should you worry? Should anybody worry? A decade ago, cholesterol was an unknown concept to most Americans; now boxes and bottles on every supermarket shelf sport "No Cholesterol" flags, and people talk of "good cholesterol" and "bad cholesterol" at parties. A recent campaign, pegged to the journalist Thomas J. Moore's new book *Heart Failure,* claims that danger of an elevated cholesterol level is largely a myth invented by American doctors intent on diagnosing a disease you probably don't have and treating you for it with expensive and dangerous drugs. This article is meant to answer these contentions, and to provide some basic information on the subject of cholesterol.

What is cholesterol? Cholesterol, a white, waxy fat known as a lipid, is an essential element in your body. Indeed all animal life requires it. It's the building block from which your body manufactures some hormones, and it's a critical component of all cell membranes. Your liver manufactures sufficient cholesterol for your body's needs every day; whatever cholesterol you eat is simply added to your overall cholesterol level. When cholesterol becomes a problem, it is usually because your diet leaves a cholesterol surplus in your bloodstream.

What's the connection between cholesterol and heart disease? For over 100 years scientists have known that cholesterol can accumulate in coronary arteries, reducing the flow of blood to the heart and eventually narrowing the passage so severely that a heart attack occurs. This process begins early in life. According to Dr. Harlan F. Weisman of Johns Hopkins, this build up, known as atherosclerotic plaque, is similar to a tumor—composed of cholesterol, fibrous tissue, and cells from the arterial wall—that encroaches on blood flow.

Whatever the critics may tell you, this is *not* theory, but fact. Among other studies, the ongoing Framingham Heart Study, begun in this Massachusetts community in 1948, clearly demonstrated that the risk of coronary artery disease (CAD) rose steadily as blood cholesterol levels rose. This link was strongest for men between 40 and 59, but not limited to them. Furthermore, studies in other countries have shown that people with high blood cholesterol levels have the most heart attacks. Finland, for example, has the highest national average of cholesterol levels and one of the highest rates of CAD; the U.S. is not far behind.

Other factors besides cholesterol may contribute to the build up of arterial plaque: smoking, elevated blood pressure, diabetes, being overweight, and a sedentary lifestyle. In addition, a family history of heart attack at an early age raises the risk of CAD. The hereditary factor is the only one that can't be significantly altered (however, even diabetes that is well-controlled may not reduce CAD risk).

What about women? Though some women under 50 do suffer from CAD, a pre-menopausal woman's risk is far less than a man's, presumably because estrogen somehow protects against the accumulation of arterial plaque. After menopause, when levels of estrogen fall, women apparently enter the same risk category as men (estrogen supplements may reduce this risk). It's true that CAD researchers have studied women much less intensively than men. But until more research has been done on women (a large study is currently being undertaken by the National Heart, Lung, and Blood Institute), it surely makes sense to assume that arterial plaque formation is as dangerous for women as for men, so women ought to follow similar advice.

What about people over 60? As with women, people 60 and older have mostly been excluded from treatment studies, so the evidence isn't as compelling. Obviously, the earlier you begin reducing your risk factors for CAD, the better off you'll be. That's why a national education program is underway, so that even small children can learn how good eating and exercise habits pay off over a lifetime.

Cholesterol may not, in fact, be the most important CAD risk factor for people over 60. However, research such as the Framingham Study clearly shows that older people with high cholesterol levels have an increased risk of CAD. If you have no symptoms of heart disease, you may wonder about the necessity of changing the way you live. But look at it this way: If you're healthy at age 60 and beyond, it's still important to safeguard the good health you have—to stop smoking, to lose weight, to consider adopting at least a modified heart-healthy diet. And it's by no means too late to take corrective measures if your blood cholesterol levels are high. Healthy habits can keep the blockage from getting worse. A recent study at U.C.L.A. suggested that it can even be reduced in some cases, albeit by drastic changes in lifestyle. Although done in a younger age group, studies have also shown that for those with elevated readings, a 1% reduction in total cholesterol translates to a 2% reduction in heart attack risk.

What if my cholesterol is the "good" kind? A determination of your LDL cholesterol and HDL cholesterol—commonly known as "bad" and "good" cholesterol—may be part of your cholesterol check. These substances, known as lipoproteins, play an important role in cholesterol transport. Just as oil and water don't mix, neither cholesterol nor any other fat is soluble in water or in blood plasma, the fluid portion of blood. Therefore, the liver puts cholesterol, other fats, and protein together in "packages" known as lipoproteins to transport them to the cells. Lipoproteins come in different sizes and composition. LDL (low-density lipoprotein) carries cholesterol to the cells. HDL (high-density lipoprotein) returns it to the liver for further processing and excretion. If your level of LDL is very high, the excess cholesterol can be deposited in the cells lining your blood vessels. A high HDL may help by removing excess cholesterol from the blood vessels. But remember: an elevated HDL may not be fully protective if your LDL levels are also high, since

an elevated LDL is an independent risk factor for CAD.

How can I lower my cholesterol with diet? Dietary cholesterol comes only from meats and animal products. No food from plants contains any cholesterol. But even the leanest animal tissue has some, as do egg yolks, milk, and other dairy products such as cheese and butter. When you eat these foods, their cholesterol is added to your own. But dietary cholesterol isn't the whole story. Fatty meats and whole-milk dairy products also contain large amounts of saturated fats ("saturated" refers to the fat's chemical structure), as do a few vegetable oils such as coconut, palm, and palm kernel oil. Hydrogenated oils, such as those in solid margarine and shortenings, are originally unsaturated fats which have been partly converted chemically to saturated fats. For reasons not completely understood, saturated fats reduce your liver's ability to remove cholesterol from the blood. Thus, it is certainly as important to lower your intake of saturated fats as to lower your intake of cholesterol. Unsaturated fats (vegetable oils such as corn, safflower, and olive are high in these) do not increase blood cholesterol and even appear to lower it.

What about drugs? Drugs exist that can reduce blood cholesterol. But they are not a magic bullet, and cannot substitute for diet and other measures to control risk factors. Many of the drugs have unpleasant side effects. While some have been in use for as long as 35 years with no evidence of long-term adverse effects, the same cannot yet be said for the newer drugs. If you have very high cholesterol, and a cholesterol-lowering diet hasn't worked, you should certainly discuss drug therapy with your doctor. Some doctors are less inclined to prescribe drugs to those over 60. However, if drugs are the only available alternative to a heart attack, they are obviously worth trying, so you might want to seek a second opinion. For most people though, a cholesterol-lowering diet is enough to bring about significant improvements.

What do the numbers mean?

Analysis of your blood cholesterol reading, now a routine part of most physical exams, is a complex matter and should be discussed with your doctor, but here are some guidelines. The first number you'll hear is your total cholesterol in milligrams per deciliter (mg/dl). As cholesterol readings can vary even from reliable labs, your doctor should advise redoing the test if your reading is high.

What to do if your blood cholesterol level is:

1. Desirable: 200 mg/dl or less.
- Plan to repeat the test in five years.
- Evaluate your other risk factors (smoking, elevated blood pressure, diabetes, severe obesity) with your doctor and take steps to control them.
2. Borderline high: 200–239 mg/dl.
- If at low risk (no history of CAD and fewer than two risk factors, one of which is being male), plan to repeat the test annually.
- If at high risk (a history of angina or a previous heart attack *or* two other CAD risk factors), *ask* for an analysis of your LDL and HDL levels.

- Take steps to modify your CAD risk factors.
- Take dietary measures to reduce your cholesterol.
3. High: 240 mg/dl or higher.
- Ask for an analysis of your LDL and HDL levels.
- Take steps to modify your CAD risk factors.
- Take dietary measures to reduce your cholesterol.
- If diet, conscientiously adhered to for six months, fails to reduce your cholesterol sufficiently, discuss drug therapy with your doctor.

Analysis of your LDL and HDL levels can change your cholesterol picture. Since LDL carries cholesterol into your arteries, and HDL picks it up for disposal, the ratio of HDL to LDL is important. Basically, the higher your HDL and the lower your LDL, the better off you are. Here's how LDL levels are classified:

- Desirable: below 130 mg/dl
- Borderline high: 130–160 mg/dl
- High: 160 mg/dl or higher

Source: *The Johns Hopkins Medical Letter,* January 1990.

---

of evidence from studies in humans and laboratory animals shows that diets low in saturated fatty acids and cholesterol are associated with low risks and rates of atherosclerotic cardiovascular diseases" (12). The health agencies of Canada and most European countries have also issued national guidelines recommending a low-fat diet.

A large amount of evidence links cancers of the breast, prostate, colon, and uterus with a high-fat intake (13). All fats are the problem here. Some scientists theorize that too many polyunsaturated fats may allow greater entry of carcinogens (cancer-initiating substances) into cells (14). Hydrogenated vegetable fats found in vegetable shortenings, margarines, and many processed foods may also contribute to cancer risk because they contain unusual **transfatty acids** created during hydrogenation (15). The American Cancer Society and the National Cancer Institute recommend we reduce intake of fats to reduce cancer risk.

Transfatty acids: "Mirror image" molecules produced during the hydrogenation of unsaturated fatty acids.

SUMMARY

Both proteins and fats are essential to health. Although many countries see severe protein malnutrition among their peoples, in the industrialized countries we consume more of these substances than we need. A high consumption of protein foods and fat can stress the body's ability to handle these substances and contribute to development of degenerative diseases such as cancer, heart disease, kidney disease and osteoporosis. Use the self-assessment exercise on page 34 to look at your own diet. If you find it too high in animal foods or fat, replace some servings with complex carbohydrate foods, such as grains, cereals, legumes, fruits, and vegetables. W

Cutting fat out of the American diet has seemingly emerged atop the agenda of America's national concerns. The American Cancer Society and the National Cancer Institute believe cutting fat intake lowers cancer risk. The American Heart Association says reducing dietary fat is an important step toward lowering heart disease risk. Now the U.S. Department of Agriculture says that fat calories are actually more fattening than carbohydrate calories.

Ways to Consume Less Fat: Foods that Do the Job

Experts believe a person reaps the most health benefits from diets containing less than 30% of their calories as fat. Some experts believe that 20% would be even better. The tips below will aid the downward descent to lowfat healthful eating.

1. Eat red meat no more than once a day. One three-ounce serving provides about 11% of the Recommended Dietary Allowance for iron and 31% for zinc while keeping fat to a minimum.
2. Choose select grades of beef instead of the more fat-marbled cuts like choice or prime.
3. Use fat-free powdered milk to lighten coffee instead of cream or non-dairy creamers.
4. Use non-stick frying pans and non-stick vegetable sprays for pan frying.
5. Remove the skin from poultry before cooking. Fat lies just under the skin.
6. To reduce oil in fried foods, drain them on a paper towel before serving.
7. Wait until oil in the pan gets hot before frying or sautéing foods. Foods soak up cold oil quicker than hot.

8. Make stews and soups containing meats the day before and refrigerate. Skim off the hardened fat before reheating.

9. Try using vegetable purees over meats, potatoes and rice instead of rich cream sauces and gravies.

10. Steer clear of high-fat snacks like potato chips and nuts. Try pretzels and hot-air popped popcorn instead.

11. Keep butter and margarine use to a minimum. They both provide about 11 grams of fat per tablespoon.

12. Add a little plain non-fat yogurt to mayonnaise. It will cut the fat without taking away the flavor.

13. Avoid cream soups. Stick to clear consommé or broth with noodles or vegetables. Eaten before a meal they may help curb appetite as well as cut fat.

14. Choose white poultry meat over dark. It contains less fat.

15. Use "diet" margarine and "diet" mayonnaise instead of the regular varieties. They cut calories and fat by one-half.

16. Limit packaged luncheon meats to sliced turkey breast and turkey pastrami.

17. Don't buy packaged foods that contain more than three grams of fat per 100 calories. Check nutrition labeling on the package to be sure.

18. Try sprinkle-on butter alternatives for hot foods. They contain only 4 calories per ½ teaspoon. One-half teaspoon of the sprinkle equals one tablespoon of butter (100 calories).

19. Choose 1% milkfat cottage cheese. Only 11% of calories come from fat, compared to regular cottage cheese which has 40% of calories from fat.

20. Avoid fast foods. Burgers, shakes and french fries are oozing with fat.

Source: *Environmental Nutrition,* March 1989.

Foods That Provide 30% or Less Calories From Fat

Beans—dried
Beef, top round—lean meat only
Breads and rolls—except
    croissant
Buttermilk
Cabbage
Cake—angel food
Cereals—most breakfast, except
    granola
Chicken breast—without skin
Cod
Cottage cheese—1 or 2%
    milkfat
Flounder
Fruits
Lentils
Peas—dried
Scallops
Snapper
Sole
Shrimp
Skim milk
Sorbet, fruit
Oysters
Tuna—packed in water
Veal, shoulder—lean meat only
Vegetables
Yogurt, frozen low-fat
Yogurt, non-fat

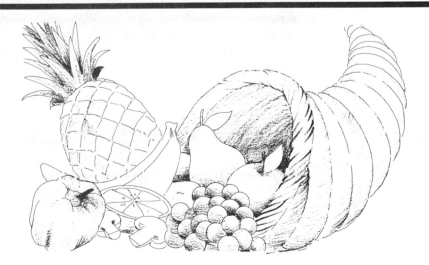

Game Plan For A Healthy Diet

Water • Vitamins • Minerals

ALTHOUGH WE APPEAR to be fairly solid, our insides are actually an internal sea. Our bodies are about two-thirds water, with a mix of minerals and organic compounds floating within. Men, because of their greater muscle mass (which contains a large amount of water), are 65 to 75 percent water. Women, who have more fat and less muscle tissue than men, are 55 to 65 percent water. This adds up to 40 to 50 quarts of water in an adult.

WATER: THE FORGOTTEN NUTRIENT

Most nutrients can be absent from the diet for several weeks or months before severe deficiency symptoms appear, yet we cannot survive without water for even a few days. Water serves as a solvent that allows the highways of the blood and **lymphatic system** to carry nutrients, oxygen, and waste. Inside cells, water is the medium in which all reactions take place. Water is the primary ingredient in digestive juices, water lubricates joints, and water acts as a natural air conditioner to regulate body temperature. This last function is one with which we are all familiar. On a hot day or during exercise, the buildup of heat in internal organs and muscles is transferred to surrounding fluids. The heat is then carried out of the body as warm sweat (even when not visibly perspiring, we lose water through our skin).

During prolonged physical activity or exposure in a hot climate, adequate water must be present to make sweat or the body overheats and heatstroke results. This is why fluid consumption is so critical for athletes—if the athlete is dehydrated, performance is impaired and risk for heatstroke is greatly increased.

Lymphatic system: A network of vessels and ducts that transport and hold fluid in the interstitial space, the area between blood vessels and cells.

(continued on p. 108)

"You are what you eat" might well be "You are what you drink." The reason is that the body is one half to two thirds water, and without taking in enough fluids you would become gravely ill within a matter of days. That's particularly important to keep in mind during the hot summer months, when we lose more water than usual through perspiration and thereby run a higher risk of suffering the chills, dizziness, nausea, and headaches brought on by dehydration.

Thirsty or Not, Drink More Fluids

Thirst, the brain's signal that the body's water level has fallen too low, goes a long way in saying we need to replace lost fluids. But those who increase their amount of physical activity in the summer through outdoor sports or exercise, which many individuals wisely do, should not rely on thirst alone as a guide for how much to drink. That's because the thirst mechanism is considerably blunted during and after vigorous activity. Older people also appear to be less likely to feel thirsty when they need water; the thirst mechanism simply becomes less efficient as we age. Moreover, aging decreases the kidney's ability to hold on to water when the body starts to become "dry," leaving elderly people especially susceptible to dehydration.

What to do? The solution is simple: Drink at least six to eight cups of fluids a day whether you feel like it or not. Water, juice, and milk will do fine. Alcoholic beverages, however, as well as the caffeine in coffee, tea, and cola drinks increase water output and thereby *raise* fluid needs, so they should not be considered as part of the six-to-eight-cup count.

"Sports drinks" touted as specially designed to restore the electrolytes sodium and potassium that are lost during exercise are not a better fluid replacement either. It's true that small amounts of sodium and potassium are lost in sweat when you exercise. However, the average American consumes 10 to 60 times the sodium he needs and enough potassium as well. All that the "special electrolytes" in these drinks actually do is cause the fluid to be absorbed less quickly from the stomach than plain water.

Six to eight cups, incidentally, is not enough to fully replace the two and a half to three quarts of fluid we lose a day. But, not to worry. The rest is supplied by "solid" food, which contains plenty of water on its own. Most fruits and vegetables, in fact, are more than 80 percent water. Water also makes up more than 50 percent of meat. Even "dry" bread is up to a third water by weight.

Source: *Tufts University Diet & Nutrition Letter,* Vol. 6, No. 5, July 1988.

Did You Know That . . .

Splashing water on yourself may make you feel refreshed, but it doesn't put water back into your system lost to perspiration, and doesn't do much to lower your body temperature.

A sedentary adult will take in and excrete 2 to 3 quarts of water a day. Water is lost primarily through urine, feces, perspiration, breath, and the skin. A loss of even 5 percent of body water results in muscle weakness and shrunken skin and a loss of 15 percent is generally fatal.

About 1 quart of the fluid lost daily is replaced through foods. Even foods that don't seem watery contain a surprising amount. Beef, for example, is 55 percent water, bread is 30 percent, vegetables are 90 percent, and cooked beans and cereals are 70 percent water. The rest of the fluid lost daily needs to be replaced by drinking water and other beverages, approximately 6 to 8 cups daily (1). Adults in the United States consume only about half this amount, an average 3 cups a day (2).

Water and Exercise

Athletes and physically active people have a special need for water, because sweat losses are high, temperature regulation is crucial, and the heart and muscles can only perform at optimal levels if enough water is present.

The critical importance of water in endurance activities became apparent to the Swiss team that made an early attempt to climb Mount Everest. Their unsuccessful effort was attributed to the fact they brought only enough fuel to melt snow for 1 pint of water per day for each man during the final days of their ascent. They became severely dehydrated and fatigued and were forced to descend. Later, Sir Edmund Hilary's team increased their fuel to allow 7 pints of water daily for each climber, and they reached the top successfully (3).

On a warm day a runner can lose 3 to 4 quarts of sweat (6 to 8 pounds) during a marathon. This fluid needs to be replaced at intervals during and after the race. During days or weeks of training, special attention must be paid to fluid intake so that sweat losses are conscientiously replaced. Athletes and coaches should monitor weight before and after workouts to estimate fluid loss and replacement needs. For every pound lost, a pint of fluid is needed to replace it. After a race or athletic event, it can take up to 24 hours of replacing fluids before the body returns to a normal hydrated state (4).

How Safe Is Our Water?

The diminishing quality of our drinking water has become a major environmental concern, rated second on the Environmental Protection Agency's list of priorities. Although community water supplies are made safe from bacterial and viral contamina-

(continued on p. 110)

When you exercise intensely, you need to replace fluids lost through sweating—particularly in hot weather, when you can easily lose more than a quart of water in an hour. At the very least, neglecting to compensate for fluid loss can cause lethargy and nausea, interfering with your performance. In endurance activities like marathon running, long-distance cycling, or even strenuous hiking, water loss can be severe, potentially producing heat exhaustion or heat stroke.

Drink to Win

What should you drink when working out? Most exercise physiologists have recommended water as the ideal replacement fluid because it is absorbed more efficiently than any other beverage. Over the past several years, though, specially formulated sports drinks such as Gatorade and Quickick have been widely touted as providing additional benefits. These drinks promise to replace the sodium and potassium lost in sweating as well as supply carbohydrates—in the form of sugar—for energy. However, in a number of studies, researchers found that sugar significantly slowed the body's absorption of fluid from the digestive tract. As a result, experts in the past consistently cautioned that beverages containing more than 2.5% sugar may hamper performance, particularly in hot weather. Most sports drinks have a sugar content of 6 to 8%; the sugar content of fruit juices and soft drinks is even higher.

Now recent research indicates that sports drinks may work as efficiently as plain water. By using new monitoring techniques to trace what happens to the fluids athletes drink, exercise physiologists at the University of South Carolina's Exercise Physiology Laboratory in Columbia discovered that although a drink containing 6% sugar may leave the stomach more slowly than water, it gets into the bloodstream just as quickly through the small intestine. Moreover, subjects performing endurance exercise experienced significantly less fatigue when they consumed the carbohydrate solution than when they drank plain water.

Other studies suggest that running and other activities that jostle the abdomen may also help force fluids through the stomach—so that, in fact, the rate at which the fluid leaves the stomach may not begin to diminish until its sugar concentration rises above 8%.

The companies that produce sports drinks have cited these studies to suggest that their products are superior to water for fluid replacement. But unless you are engaging in *long work-outs, there is no evidence that sports drinks offer any advantage over water.* In virtually all of these studies the subjects were trained endurance athletes who exercised two hours or more, and the researchers noted that sports drinks will probably not provide any benefit over water during shorter bouts of exercise. In hot weather, furthermore, replacing fluid is far more critical than restoring carbohydrates (which you can obtain by eating crackers or other high-carbohydrate foods) or sodium (easily replaced through your normal diet).

The researchers also point out that the efficiency of any fluid varies tremendously among individuals. Some people's systems don't handle sports drinks well, so that even when the drinks are diluted they may cause nausea. Nor has any one type of carbohydrate drink proven superior. Ads for glucose polymer drinks such as Exceed, which contain chains of glucose molecules, have claimed that these beverages enter the bloodstream faster than other drinks containing high concentrations of simple glucose and/or sucrose. But studies comparing sports drinks have found no significant difference in their rate of absorption.

If you want to spend the money on sports drinks, that's up to you. If a sports drink makes you feel bloated, try diluting it with one to three parts water—or switch completely to water.

Whatever you drink . . .

The most important thing is to drink, period—even if you don't feel thirsty. Thirst is satisfied long before you have replenished lost fluids. Research shows that cool drinks (40° to 50°) are absorbed more quickly than lukewarm ones. In hot weather drink at least 16 to 20 ounces of fluid two hours before exercising and another 8 ounces 15 to 30 minutes before. While you exercise drink 3 to 7 ounces every 10 to 20 minutes. After exercising, drink enough to replace the fluid you've sweated off (weigh yourself before and after your workout; drink one pint for each pound lost) and eat normally.

Source: *University of California Berkeley Wellness Letter,* August 1989.

tion through filtering and chlorination, industrial and agricultural pollution results in toxic heavy metals, cancer-causing organic chemicals, nitrates, pesticides, and asbestos that increasingly find their way in. The Environmental Protection Agency has found 1000 contaminants in the nation's water supply, but has set enforceable limits for only 30 of these (5). And although chlorine kills microorganisms in water, a study by the National Cancer Institute in 1987 concluded the chemical may be contributing to bladder cancer (6).

Many people are using home filtration systems because of concern about water safety, but tests show these are not problem-free. Some are ineffective and others encourage the growth of microorganisms (7). The concern about pure water has resulted in over 700 brands of bottled water becoming available (8). In 1987, Americans in 1 out of every 6 households bought an estimated 1.25 billion gallons of bottled water for a total cost of $1.5 billion (5). Many brands are simply from the tap of another locality and may be no better or worse than your local water. In fact, bottled water must only be monitored for 22 contaminants, whereas community water supplies are monitored for an additional 8, according to the Center for Science in the Public Interest (5). Some bottled waters contain large amounts of minerals. These too are not necessarily good for us. Water high in minerals can disrupt the body's normal balance of minerals, and water containing large amounts of sodium is unwise for people with sodium-sensitive high blood pressure.

For the health-conscious individual, obtaining clean, pure water appears a pursuit fraught with trade-offs and unknowns; the dilemma will not go away until as communities and as a nation we face the problems engendered by the technology of our industrial and agricultural methods.

Game Strategy: Fluids

Surprisingly, the sensation of thirst is inaccurate in guiding our fluid intake to meet optimal levels. In physically active people and the elderly, research has shown the thirst signal underestimates fluid needs by about one-third (9). In addition, the average person underconsumes fluids (2). This means most people must make a conscious effort to drink enough even when thirst is not felt. For a sedentary person, 6 to 8 glasses of fluids a day are adequate, but the exerciser will need more.

One method of estimating fluid needs for physically active people is based on caloric intake: Drink 1 quart for every 1000 calories consumed daily. For an athlete eating 6000 calories a day, then, 6 quarts of fluid are needed (10).

Many commonly consumed beverages contain the **diuretic** substances caffeine or alcohol. Coffee, black tea, caffeinated soft drinks, wine, beer, and other alcoholic drinks cause some water to be drawn out of cells and urination to increase. Don't count these as contributing toward fluid intake.

If you need to increase your fluid intake, take advantage of drinking fountains, keep a bottle of water on your desk, carry water with you on bike rides and outings, and make a habit of having a glass of water, juice, or other caffeine and alcohol-free beverage next to you when you read or watch TV.

VITAMINS: TRUE TEAM PLAYERS

Vitamins are potent organic (carbon-containing) molecules needed in very small amounts in the diet. They cannot be manufactured by the body. The amount we need each day totals less than one-

Diuretic: A compound that stimulates increased excretion of water via the kidneys.

(continued on p. 115)

Water: Safe to Swallow?

If all the water on earth could fit in a gallon jug, and if you poured out the portion that was non-drinkable (too salty, polluted, or hard to get), you'd end up with one single drop. Is that drop safe to drink? Not if you happened to be in Des Moines, Iowa on September 27, 1983. On that day, levels of trichloroethylene (TCE)—a suspected carcinogen—soared to more than 18 times the current federal limit. In fact, throughout the late 70s and early 80s, the 190,000 residents of Des Moines routinely drank water with anywhere from two to ten times the amount of TCE now permitted.

How did this hazardous solvent get into the municipal water system? A local company used it in the 1960s to remove grease from metal wheels and brakes. The firm disposed of the oily waste by spraying some of it on the parking lot (for "dust control") and by dumping the rest into a nearby drainage ditch.

Now *your* water might not be as bad as Des Moines' was. Then again . . .

The sad truth is that your drinking water could contain any of nearly 1,000 contaminants. Sadder yet, the Environmental Protection Agency (EPA) has set enforceable limits for just 30 of the 1,000. (There was none for TCE back in 1983.) What's more, many of those 30 limits were established years ago, and are considered too high by today's standards.

Consider The Source. Rivers, lakes, and reservoirs supply about half the population, including most major cities. On the way to the purification plant, this "surface" water can pick up some unsavory companions: pollutants from industrial discharges, mining wastes, pesticide runoff from farms or roads.

The rest of us drink "ground" water, which comes from slow-moving, underground "rivers" that feed our wells and springs. Ground water supplies 97 percent of all rural households, portions of about 20 major cities (including Los Angeles, New York, and Spokane), and most of Florida. It can become contaminated from leak-ing municipal landfills, underground gasoline storage tanks, hazardous waste storage or disposal sites, or septic tanks.

Meet The Pollutants. The list of 1,000 contaminants identified by the EPA reads like a *Who's Who* of environmental pollutants: bacteria, benzene, lead, mercury, PCBs.

Some of the 1,000 even come from our attempts to purify the water supply. Surface water often contains decaying leaves or other plant or animal matter. When this water is treated with chlorine (as nearly all surface water is), cancer-causing compounds can form.

In 1987, a major study by the National Cancer Institute (NCI)[1] concluded that the risk of developing bladder cancer rose with increased intake of beverages made with chlorinated surface water—which is what comes out of the tap in about half the households in the U.S.

"We estimate that chlorinated surface water is responsible for about a quarter of all bladder cancer cases among non-smokers, if the relationship is causal," says study co-author Robert Hoover.

Bladder cancer primarily affects the elderly, and is the fifth most common cancer in the U.S. Its incidence has increased by more than 50 percent since 1950.

The NCI is now looking for a link between chlorinated surface water and other types of cancer—something the first study wasn't designed to detect.

Get The Lead Out. Both surface and ground water can pick up an unwanted passenger on the trip from the purification plant to the tap: lead.

Lead can raise blood pressure, cause babies to be born premature or underweight, and impair the mental abilities of children. The Centers for Disease Control estimated that 10.4 million children in the U.S. are exposed to significant amounts of lead in their drinking water.

"The more we learn about lead, the more we find adverse effects at lower and lower levels," says Joel Schwartz, senior scientist at the EPA. "Drinking water is now a major source of lead for a sizable portion of the population. It's a matter of considerable concern."

If your home has lead pipes, or has copper pipes with lead solder that were installed less than five years ago *and* your water is acidic, you could be ingesting high levels of lead. The only way to know for sure is to have your water tested.

Meanwhile, minimize exposure by sticking to the "C" tap for drinking and cooking (let it run until it gets as cold as it's going to, which could take a few minutes if you haven't used any water or flushed a toilet for several hours).

EPA To The Rescue? The EPA requires your utility to keep your water below the Maximum Contaminant Levels (MCLs) for just 30 potential pollutants.

In 1986 Congress ordered the EPA to increase the number of regulated contaminants from 30 to 83 by June of 1989. Needless to say, things are already behind schedule.

"I just can't believe how little the EPA has accomplished in the last 14 years," says Ned Groth, associate technical director of Consumers Union.

The National Wildlife Federation (NWF) goes even further. A report released in early October charges that "millions of Americans are drinking unsafe water."[2]

The NWF claims that public water systems committed more than 100,000 violations of the Safe Drinking Water Act in 1987. What's more, says the environmental group, the water utilities broke the law "94 percent of the time," by failing to inform consumers when violations occurred.

Your Right To Know Your water provider must give you the results of its testing . . . if you ask. This will cover the 30 contaminants that are regulated, up to 36 others that must (eventually) be monitored, plus any additional ones your state requires.

Once you know *how much* of *what* is in your water, find out how much is *too much,* by calling the EPA Safe Drinking Water Hotline at (800) 426-4791 (382-5533 in Washington, D.C.). Ask for a list of finalized and proposed federal standards

as well as any "health advisories" or guidelines for contaminants that have no standards.

Pay particular attention to the level of "total trihalomethanes" (THMs), which are the contaminants most clearly related to your risk of developing bladder cancer. According to the National Academy of Sciences, the EPA's standard of 100 micrograms per liter (mcg/l, or ppb) is too high.[3] We suggest a level of 10 mcg/l.

Testing, Testing. You should consider going through the expense of testing your tap water if:

- You drink from your own well or other private water supply.
- You notice a change in your water's color, taste, or odor. (Some utilities will do free sampling at your tap.)
- You suspect the presence of lead. (Make sure the lab can detect levels down to 10 parts per billion.)
- Your water company serves fewer than 3,300 people. If so, it doesn't have to comply with new monitoring requirements as quickly as larger systems.
- You live near a hazardous waste dump, industrial park, chemical manufacturing plant, military base, or non-organic farm.

If you decide to test, call the EPA Safe Drinking Water Hotline for the name of the drinking water laboratory certification officer for your state. He or she should be able to give you a list of approved labs.

Since there are hundreds of potential pollutants, try to narrow the field before testing. Under the Emergency Planning and Community Right-To-Know Law, you can obtain information about hazardous chemicals (but not pesticides) in your community. *Using Community Right-to-Know: A Guide to A New Federal Law* is available for $5.00 from OMB Watch, 2001 "O" St., N.W., Washington, D.C. The EPA Emergency Planning & Community Right-to-Know Hotline, at (800) 535-0202 (479-2449 in Washington D.C.), also provides information. For pesticide questions, call your local agricultural extension agent.

Is Your Water Radioactive?

It's entirely possible . . . if you drink ground water that has passed through granite or other uranium-containing rocks. And if your water *is* radioactive, chances are it's contaminated by radon, which is a byproduct of uranium decay.

"The risk from radon in drinking water is larger than the risk from everything else the EPA regulates in drinking water combined," says Douglas Crawford-Brown, professor at the School of Public Health at the University of North Carolina at Chapel Hill.

Drinking radon-tainted water probably poses little threat to your health. But radon in your water becomes radon in your air every time you turn on the shower. And breathing radon can be deadly.

The EPA estimates that anywhere from 5,000 to 20,000 lung cancer deaths in the U.S. each year are attributable to the radioactive gas.

Many people believe they don't have to test for radon if they live above the second floor. But if you live in an area with high concentrations of radon in drinking water (New England, the Rocky Mountains, the southern Appalachians), you should probably set up a test in your bathroom, no matter what floor you live on. "EPA listed" radon testing kits can be obtained for less than $10 in many supermarkets.

What's a safe radon level? The EPA says the goal for your home should be no more than 4 picocuries per liter (pC/l) of air. But at that level, your lifetime risk of dying of lung cancer is between 1-in-100 and 5-in-100. That's roughly equivalent to smoking half a pack of cigarettes a day, which is clearly too high. A better goal is 1 pC/l, which is the average indoor radon level in homes across the country.

Home Treatment. Home filters can make a difference . . . if you know how to select and maintain them. If you don't, they can actually *increase* contaminant levels.

A good overview of existing systems can be found in *Is Your Water Safe To Drink?* by Raymond Gabler and the editors of Consumer Report Books (available in major bookstores).

Is Bottled Better? If sales figures were synonymous with health value, bottled water would be as pure as the TV commercials suggest.

Americans spent $1.5 billion on an estimated 1.25 billion gallons of bottled water in 1987, according to the International Bottled Water Association (IBWA). "One out of six households now uses bottled water as its primary source of drinking water," says IBWA executive vice president William Deal. The industry group claims that in California the figure is one out of three.

The IBWA is careful not to make any health claims for bottled water, but it's clear that the industry profits from the perception that bottled is better.

Is it?

As far as federal authorities are concerned, bottled water currently has to meet standards for only 22 contaminants: *eight fewer than for tap water.* And, the Food and Drug Administration doesn't even have a monitoring program to see if that's being done.

"If no one looks, no one finds," says Sandra Marquardt of Greenpeace, co-author of a forthcoming Environmental Policy Institute report on bottled water.

Mineral and soda waters, which are used by millions of people as their main source of drinking water, don't even have to meet the same quality standards as other bottled water.

- A 1987 state survey revealed that 13 of 15 brands of mineral water sold in Massachusetts exceeded one or more federal or state guidelines.
- A New York survey found traces of toluene, carbon tetrachloride, and other solvents in 48 of 93 bottled waters sampled last year.
- A British study found high levels of bacteria in 20 of 29 non-carbonated mineral waters.[4]

- Researchers at Northeastern University discovered several kinds of antibiotic-resistant bacteria in 6 of 8 brands of bottled spring and distilled water purchased in the Boston area.[5]

Not only is bottled less regulated than tap; sometimes bottled *is* tap. "Drinking water" on the label probably means tap water inside bottle. The tap also can provide the raw material for "purified," "distilled," "soda," "club," and even some "mineral" waters. The exception is "spring" water, which should come from an underground source. But even that's no guarantee of purity.

So is bottled better? Some probably is . . . and some definitely isn't.

One thing you can do is ask the bottler for the latest test results for *all* the chemicals it checks for. Then compare the numbers to the standards or guidelines you get by calling the EPA hotline.

You might or might not learn something. Poland Spring sent us test results for only 15 contaminants, Great Bear gave us 17, Evian sent 24, and Mountain Valley sent 51. After some convincing, Perrier gave us test results for 93 contaminants. It normally sends 12. None of the contaminant levels provided by the bottlers exceeded federal standards.

What It All Boils Down To. There is no clear winner in the Water Derby. Tap, filtered, or bottled—each has its own risks.

Even boiling regular tap water (which kills germs) can end up concentrating the contaminants it doesn't remove.

One safe (but not particularly palate-pleasing) choice is to boil distilled water. Distillation gets rid of chemicals with a boiling point greater than water, while boiling takes care of most of the rest, as well as bacteria and other biological contaminants.

It's not going to win any taste tests, but you probably won't notice the difference if you use it to make juice or tea.

And since distilled water has no minerals, you should be particularly careful to eat foods rich in calcium and magnesium (dairy products, whole grains, and vegetables).

—Lisa Lefferts and Stephen B. Schmidt

1. *J. Nat. Cancer Inst. 79:* 1269, 1987.
2. National Wildlife Federation (Washington, D.C.), *Danger on Tap,* 1988.
3. National Academy of Sciences (Washington, D.C.), *Drinking Water and Health: 7,* 1987.
4. *Epid. Infec 99:* 439, 1987.
5. *Can. J. Microbiol. 33:* 286, 1987.

Source: *Nutrition Action Healthletter,* November 1988, pp. 1, 5–7.

---

eighth of a teaspoon, yet without them health and mental functioning would be severely impaired and death would follow.

Unlike the energy nutrients (proteins, fats, and carbohydrates), vitamins are not used as fuel or building materials. Their role lies solely in regulating and facilitating the millions of chemical reactions that take place in the body. They remain unchanged in the process and are able to carry on their function repeatedly. Without a given vitamin, the particular reactions it governs cannot take place. For example, without vitamin D, calcium will not be placed into the bone structure even though adequate calcium is available. Without certain B vitamins, the calories in carbohydrates remain "locked up," unable to be used for fuel, and energy for bodily functions suffers.

Vitamins are divided into two major categories, those that are fat-soluble and found in the fatty portions of food and body tissues, and those that are water-soluble, and found in the aqueous portions. Vitamins A, D, E, and K are **fat-soluble vitamins**. The eight B vitamins and vitamin C are water-soluble.

The body can store excess amounts of the fat-soluble vitamins for future use. For this reason, foods rich in these nutrients do not have to be consumed every day (although it doesn't hurt!). The **water-soluble vitamins** are far more readily excreted from the body and daily intakes of these vitamins are needed to maintain tissue levels. Consuming a wide variety of unprocessed foods is the best way to ensure an optimal vitamin intake.

A balanced nutrient supplement providing vitamins and minerals in levels at or close to the RDAs has never been shown to be harmful, although nutritionists differ in their opinions as to whether these are needed. A caution is clearly in order regarding large intakes of single vitamin supplements, however. High doses of the fat-soluble vitamins A and D can be toxic since the body has no effective way to excrete them. They build up in liver and fat

Fat-soluble vitamins:
Vitamins that are found in the fatty portions of foods and that can be stored in the body. Vitamins A, E, and D are fat-soluble.

Water-soluble vitamins:
Vitamins that are found in the watery compartments of foods and the body; excreted in the urine if body concentrations become too high. The B-complex vitamins and vitamin C are water-soluble.

"Vitamins: Try none a day." So advised a headline in one of the nation's most widely circulated newspapers, relaying what were interpreted as the latest recommendations from the National Research Council regarding nutritional supplements. Other newspapers followed suit. "Supplements said useless" and "Diet panel backs . . . no pills" are just two of the other headlines that have appeared.

No Supplements for Anyone at All?

But those messages did not tell the whole story. It's true that in its recent 1300-page report entitled *Diet and Health,* the National Research Council says that rather than taking supplements, "the desirable way for the general public to obtain recommended levels of nutrients is by eating a variety of foods." Still, the report does point out certain instances in which people might need a vitamin and/or mineral pill. Women who suffer from excessive menstrual bleeding, for example, may require iron supplements to replenish stores of that mineral lost through blood. Pregnant women as well as those who are breastfeeding may benefit from supplements too, since their needs for nutrients such as iron, folic acid, and calcium increase beyond what they may be able to obtain from food.

People who follow very low-calorie regimens along with strict vegetarians, whose diets often do not supply enough calcium, iron, zinc, or vitamin B$_{12}$, may also benefit from taking vitamin and mineral supplements. And a vitamin/mineral preparation may be in order for individuals who are suffering from diseases or taking medications that can interfere with their appetite or the way the body uses or rids itself of certain nutrients, thereby making it particularly difficult for diet alone to meet nutritional needs. Finally, newborns often need a single dose of vitamin K immediately after birth to prevent abnormal bleeding. The diets of certain groups of otherwise healthy people have also been found to fall short of adequate levels of certain nutrients. Several studies on the elderly, for example, have shown that many are eating diets low in calcium, zinc, vitamins B$_6$, B$_{12}$, D, E, and folate. And although the Research Council does not make any blanket recommendation for senior citizens, a supplement that contains more than 100 percent of the U.S. Recommended Daily Allowances for vitamins and minerals may provide those who do not eat enough or cannot shop and cook adequately with the nutrients they're missing.

Of course, none of this means that popping a vitamin or mineral pill should be viewed as a panacea for a poor diet, or that taking excess amounts of one or another nutrient is a healthy practice. Indeed, ingesting large doses of certain nutrients can cause harm. Too much vitamin A, for example, can lead to liver damage. That's one reason the report was so careful to advise Americans to "avoid taking dietary supplements in excess of the RDA in any one day."

Still, interpreting the report as advising "none a day" across the board when it comes to vitamin and mineral supplements is oversimplifying the matter. Sometimes taking *one* a day, under the guidance of a physician or dietitian, is a called-for step to take.

Source: *Tufts University Diet & Nutrition Letter,* Vol. 7, No. 4, June 1989.

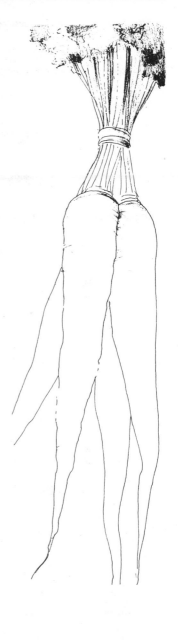

tissue and ultimately cause severe toxicity. Cases of severe vitamin A poisoning and a few fatalities occur every year in the United States among children who, perhaps, got into the chewable vitamin bottle or adults who took large amounts not understanding the risks. Even though the water-soluble vitamins can be excreted by the kidneys, excessive intakes can be harmful because levels in the blood will greatly exceed normal levels before they are excreted. For example, large doses of vitamin B$_6$ cause nerve damage; of niacin, can result in liver damage; and of vitamin C, can cause gastric upset and diarrhea (11).

Vitamins are not only necessary for life but have roles in the long-term prevention of specific diseases. Fruits and vegetables that are rich in **beta-carotene** (a compound made into vitamin A once inside the body) and in vitamin C may decrease risk of

Beta-carotene: A water-soluble compound found in fruits and vegetables that is transformed into vitamin A by the body.

(continued on p. 123)

Table 5.1 About Vitamins

Vitamin	Functions	Best Sources	Comments
Vitamin A (retinol) and beta-carotene (pro-vitamin A)	Vision, skin, bone growth, reproduction	Deep yellow and orange fruits and vegetables, dark green leafy vegetables, liver	Retinol is toxic in large doses; beta-carotene has role in cancer prevention
Vitamin D	Absorption of calcium, bone growth	Sunlight, fish liver, fortified milk	Toxic in large doses
Vitamin E	Protects cells from oxidative damage	Vegetable oils	Low toxicity
Vitamin K	Blood clotting	Leafy green vegetables	Synthesized by bacteria; deficiency rare
Vitamin C	Connective tissue synthesis	Citrus fruits, potatoes, leafy vegetables, tomatoes	Role in cancer prevention
Thiamin (Vitamin B1)	Release of energy from carbohydrate	Grains, legumes, pork	
Riboflavin (Vitamin B2)	Release of energy from protein, fat and carbohydrate	Dairy products, enriched or whole grains, organ meats, meats	Destroyed by exposure to light
Niacin	Release of energy from protein, fat and carbohydrate synthesis of protein, fat, DNA	Liver, meat, legumes, poultry, enriched or whole grains	Excessive amounts cause liver damage
Pyridoxine (Vitamin B6)	Protein synthesis, immunity	Whole grains (not enriched), meat, liver, eggs, vegetables	Deficiency most common in people whose diets are high in processed foods
Folacin	Synthesis of DNA, RNA	Green vegetables, liver, legumes, whole grains (not enriched)	Deficiency causes anemia
Vitamin B12	Aids folacin in DNA synthesis	Meat, fish, eggs, cheese, milk, liver	Deficiency causes anemia, nerve damage
Pantothenic Acid	Release of energy from fuel nutrients, synthesis of many compounds	Whole grains (not enriched), vegetables, fish, poultry, liver	Processed foods are a poor source

Vitamins are potent organic molecules. Although only very small amounts are needed, these cannot be manufactured by the body and must be provided by the diet. Consuming a wide variety of unprocessed foods is the best way to ensure an optimal vitamin intake.

Some Facts and Myths of Vitamins

Should you take vitamins or not? The question has yet to be adequately settled. Thus we offer the point of view proposed in this article by the Food and Drug Administration in deliberate contrast to that taken in the article "No Supplements for Anyone At All?" on page 116.

Vitamins are organic compounds necessary in small amounts in the diet for the normal growth and maintenance of life of animals, including man.

They do not provide energy, nor do they construct or build any part of the body. They are needed for transforming foods into energy and body maintenance. There are 13 or more of them, and if any one is missing a deficiency disease becomes apparent.

Vitamins are similar because they are made of the same elements—carbon, hydrogen, oxygen, and sometimes nitrogen. (Vitamin B_{12} also contains cobalt.) They are different in that their elements are arranged differently, and each vitamin performs one or more specific functions in the body.

At first, no one knew what vitamins were chemically, and they were identified by letters. Later, what was thought to be one vitamin turned out to be many, and numbers were added; the B complex is the best example.

Then some were found unnecessary for human needs and were removed from the list, which accounts for some of the gaps in the numbers and letters. Examples of those removed are B_8, adenylic acid; B_{13}, orotic acid; and B_{15}, pangamic acid. Others, originally designated differently, were found to be the same. For example, vitamins H, M, S, W, and X were all shown to be biotin; vitamin G became vitamin B_2 (riboflavin); and vitamin Y became B_6 (pyridoxine, pyridoxal, and pyridoxamine). Vitamin M seems to have been used for three different vitamins—folic acid, pantothenic acid, and biotin.

Extremely sensitive methods of measuring the potency or quantity of vitamins have been developed because they are present in foods in very small amounts. Some vitamins are measured in I.U.s (international units), which is a measure of biological activity. Other vitamins are expressed by weight in micrograms or milligrams.

To illustrate the small amounts needed by the human body, let's start with an ounce, which is 28.4 grams. A milligram is 1/1000 of a gram, and a microgram is 1/1000 of a milligram. The U.S. Recommended Daily Allowance (U.S. RDA) of vitamin B_{12} for an adult is 6 micrograms a day. Just one ounce of this vitamin could supply the daily needs of 4,724,921 people.

Getting enough vitamins is essential to life, although the body has no nutritional use for excess vitamins and some vitamins can be stored only for relatively short periods. Many people, nevertheless, believe in being on the "safe side" and thus take extra vitamins. However, a well-balanced diet will usually meet all the body's vitamin needs.

So-called average or normal eaters probably never need supplement vitamins, although many think they do. Vitamin deficiency diseases are rarely seen in the U.S. population. People known to have deficient diets require supplemental vitamins, as do those recovering from certain illnesses or vitamin deficiencies.

People who are interested in nutrition and good health should become familiar with the initials U.S. RDA. "United States Recommended Daily Allowances" were adopted by FDA for use in nutrition labeling and special dietary foods. They are the highest amounts of vitamins, minerals and proteins that are needed by most people each day.

The accompanying table lists the U.S. RDAs for vitamins used in nutrition labeling of foods, including foods that are also vitamin supplements.

Following is a rundown of the 13 major vitamins, how the body uses them, and what foods contain them:

Vitamin A—Retinol

Vitamin A like vitamins D, E, and K, is an oil soluble vitamin and is stored in the liver. (Generally, oil soluble vitamins can be stored for long periods—even indefinitely—in the body. Water soluble vitamins are retained for shorter periods.) This vitamin is necessary for new cell growth and healthy tissues and is essential for vision in dim light (night blindness), high sensitivity to light, and other eye maladies. Vitamin A deficiency can cause dry rough skin that may become more susceptible to infection.

Children and young people who have been given large doses of vitamin A developed an increased pressure inside the skull that mimics symptoms of a brain tumor so convincingly that in several cases hospital personnel made preparations for surgery before the high intake of vitamin A was discovered. Research with animals and some reports suggest that excess vitamin A may cause birth defects. The amount needed to cause this harm is not known. Vitamin A activity is found in foods in two forms: carotene, a yellow pigment in green and yellow vegetables and yellow fruit that the human body converts to vitamin A, and vitamin A itself, formed from carotene by other animals and stored in certain food tissues such as liver, eggs, and milk. Unlike vitamin A, carotene is virtually nontoxic.

Vitamin B$_1$—Thiamin
This vitamin is water soluble, as are all in the B complex. Thiamin is required for normal digestion, growth, fertility, lactation, the normal functioning of nerve tissue, and carbohydrate metabolism.

Vitamin B$_1$ deficiency causes beriberi, a dysfunctioning of the nervous system. Other deficiency problems are loss of appetite, body swelling (edema), heart problems, nausea, vomiting, and spastic muscle contractions.

Vitamin B$_2$—Riboflavin
Riboflavin helps the body obtain energy from carbohydrates and protein substances. A deficiency of this vitamin causes lip sores and cracks, as well as dimness of vision. Riboflavin is abundant in leafy vegetables, enriched and whole-grain breads, liver, cheese, lean meats, milk, and eggs.

Niacin
Niacin is necessary for healthy condition of all tissue cells. A Niacin deficiency causes pellagra, which once was next to rickets the most common deficiency disease in the United States. Pellagra is characterized by rough skin, mouth sores, diarrhea, and mental disorders.

Niacin is one of the most stable of the vitamins, the most easily obtained, and the cheapest. The most abundant natural sources are liver, lean meats, peas, beans, enriched and whole-grain cereal products, and fish.

Pantothenic Acid
Pantothenic acid is needed to support a variety of body functions, including proper growth and maintenance. A deficiency may cause headache, fatigue, poor muscle coordination, nausea, and cramps.

Pantothenic acid is abundant in liver, eggs, white potatoes, sweet potatoes, peas, whole-grains (particularly wheat) and peanuts.

Folic Acid (Folacin)
Folic acid helps the body to manufacture red blood cells and is essential in normal metabolism which is, basically, the conversion of foods to energy. A deficiency causes a type of anemia. The most abundant sources are liver, navy beans, and dark-green leafy vegetables. Other good sources are nuts, fresh oranges, and whole-wheat products.

Vitamin B$_6$—Pyridoxine—Pyridoxal—Pyridoxamine
Vitamin B$_6$ has three forms but all are used by the body in the same way.

This vitamin is involved mostly in the utilization of protein. As with other vitamins, B$_6$ is essential for the proper growth and maintenance of the body functions. Deficiency symptoms include mouth soreness, dizziness, nausea, and weight loss, and sometimes severe nervous disturbances.

Pyridoxine is found abundantly in liver, whole-grain cereals, potatoes, red meats, green vegetables, and yellow corn.

Vitamin B$_{12}$
Vitamin B$_{12}$ is necessary for the normal development of red blood cells, and the functioning of all cells, particularly in the bone marrow, nervous system, and intestines.

A deficiency causes pernicious anemia, and if the deficiency is prolonged, a degeneration of the spinal cord occurs.

Abundant sources are organ meats, lean meats, fish, milk, eggs, and shellfish. B_{12} is not present to any measurable degree in plants, which means that strict vegetarians should supplement their diets with this vitamin.

Biotin

Once called vitamin H, biotin is now the sole descriptive term for this vitamin, which is actually a member of the B complex. It is important in the metabolism of carbohydrates, proteins, and fats.

Most deficiency symptoms involve mild skin disorders, some anemia, depression, sleepiness, and muscle pain. A deficiency is extremely rare, probably because the bacteria in the intestinal tract produces biotin so that more is excreted than consumed in the diet.

Abundant dietary sources include eggs, milk, and meats. Raw egg white contains a factor that destroys biotin.

Vitamin C—Asorbic Acid

This least stable of the vitamins promotes growth and tissue repair, including the healing of wounds. It aids in tooth formation and bone formation. When used as a food additive, vitamin C acts as a preservative. Lack of this vitamin causes scurvy, one of the oldest diseases known to man. The signs of scurvy include lassitude, weakness, bleeding, loss of weight, and irritability. An early sign is bleeding of the gums and ease of bruising.

Abundant sources are turnip greens, green peppers, kale, broccoli, mustard greens, citrus fruits, strawberries, currants, tomatoes, and other vegetables. You can get all the vitamin C your body needs by eating daily a 3- to 4-ounce serving of any of the foods named.

Vitamin D

This vitamin also exists in several forms. The most common (and equally effective) are vitamin D_2 and vitamin D_3. The D_2 is a plant source; D_3 comes from animals.

Vitamin D aids in the absorption of calcium and phosphorus in bone formation. To accom-

plish its work, the body—through the liver and the kidneys—converts the vitamin to a hormone-like material.

Vitamin D deficiency causes rickets. The obvious signs are skeleton deformation—bowed legs, deformed spine, "pot-belly" appearance, and sometimes flat feet and stunting of growth.

Too much vitamin D can cause nausea, weight loss, weakness, excessive urination, and the more serious conditions of hypertension and calcification of soft tissues, including the blood vessels and kidneys. Bone deformities and multiple fractures are also common. In fact, many of the symptoms from an excess of vitamin D are remarkably similar to those caused by a deficiency.

Abundant sources are canned and fresh fish (particularly the salt water varieties), egg yolk, and the vitamin D-fortified foods such as milk and margarine. People who spend part of their time in the sun with exposure of the skin need no other source of vitamin D, since it is formed in the skin by the ultraviolet rays. Foods fortified with vitamin D are intended mainly for infants and the elderly who lack exposure to sunlight. The daily requirement is very small and excess amounts above that are stored in the body.

Vitamin K

There are several natural forms of vitamin K, which are essential to blood clotting. One type K_1, occurs in plants. Another, K_2, is formed by bacteria in the intestinal tract. Yet a third is found in some animals and birds. The synthetic vitamin K, menadione, because of the potential for harm involved in its use, is dispensed only by prescription. Phyloquinone, K_1, may be used in dietary supplements up to a level of 100 micrograms per recommended daily quantity.

A deficiency causes hemorrhage and liver injury. Vitamin K is found in spinach, lettuce, kale, cabbage, cauliflower, liver, and egg yolk.

Vitamin E

Vitamin E in humans acts as an antioxidant that helps to prevent oxygen from destroying other substances. In other words, vitamin E is a preservative, protecting the activity of other compounds such as vitamin A. No clinical effects have been

UNITED STATES RECOMMENDED DAILY ALLOWANCES

	Unit	Infants (0-12 mo.)	Children under 4 yrs.	Adults and children 4 or more yrs.	Pregnant or lactating women
Vitamin A	IU	1500	2500	5000	8000
Vitamin D	IU	400	400	400	400
Vitamin E	IU	5	10	30	30
Vitamin C	mg	35	40	60	60
Folacin	mg	0.1	0.2	0.4	0.8
Thiamin (B$_1$)	mg	0.5	0.7	1.5	1.7
Riboflavin (B$_2$)	mg	0.6	0.8	1.7	2.0
Niacin	mg	8	9	20	20
Vitamin B$_6$	mg	0.4	0.7	2	2.5
Vitamin B$_{12}$	mcg	2	3	6	8
Biotin	mg	0.05	0.15	0.3	0.3
Pantothenic acid	mg	3	5	10	10

IU = International unit
mg = milligram
mcg = microgram

The U.S. RDA System was developed by FDA for its nutrition labeling and dietary supplement programs. This table for use in the labeling of dietary supplements lists only vitamin requirements, for purpose of this article.

associated with very low intake of this vitamin in humans. A rather rare form of anemia in premature infants, however, responds to vitamin E medication. A diet high in polyunsaturated fat including the fish oils containing omega 3 fatty acids, requires a small increase in dietary vitamin E to prevent oxidation of this rather unstable form of fat.

Abundant sources are vegetable oils, beans, eggs, whole grains (the germ), liver, fruits, and vegetables.

Vitamin E is one of the most talked about vitamins, and to some extent the exaggerated and unsubstantiated claims made for vitamin E result from a combination of hope and misinterpretation.

The committee on Nutritional Misinformation of the National Academy of Sciences has issued a report on vitamin E. Three statements are quoted here:

"Surveys of the U.S. population indicate that the adequate amounts of vitamin E are supplied by the usual diet."

"Careful studies over a period of years attempting to relate these (test animal) symptoms to vitamin E deficiency in human beings have been unproductive."

"Self-medication with vitamin E in hope that a more or less serious condition will be alleviated may indeed be hazardous, especially when appropriate diagnosis and treatment may thereby be delayed or avoided."

Most of us view scientific knowledge with awe, and we are quite justified, considering the scientific achievements of our age. Misconceptions about vitamins and their proper functions are understandable; no primer would be complete that fails to clear up some of these misconceptions:

Myth: Vitamins give you "pep" and "energy."

Fact: Vitamins yield no calories. They, of themselves, provide no extra pep or vitality beyond normal expectations, nor do they provide unusual levels of well-being.

Myth: Timing of vitamin intake is crucial.

Fact: There is no medical or scientific basis for this contention.

Myth: Vitamins must be taken in precisely formulated amounts and ratios to each other in order to have best effects.

Fact: Intake should be adequate but not excessive for each. No precise ratios are required.

Myth: Organic or natural vitamins are nutritionally superior to synthetic vitamins.

Fact: Synthetic vitamins, manufactured in the laboratory, are identical to the natural vitamins found in foods. The body cannot tell the difference and gets the same benefits from either source. Statements to the effect that "Nature cannot be imitated" and "natural vitamins have the essence of life" are without meaning.

Myth: Vitamin C "protects" against the common cold.

Fact: Too bad, but extensive clinical research fails to support this.

Myth: The more vitamins the better.

Fact: Taking excess vitamins is a complete waste, both in money and effect. In fact, as noted, excess amounts of any of several different vitamins can be harmful.

Myth: You cannot get enough vitamins from the conventional foods you eat.

Fact: Anyone who eats a reasonably varied diet should normally never need supplemental vitamins.

Source: U.S. Department of Health and Human Services, Public Health Service, *FDA Consumer* HHS Publication No. (FDA) 88-2117, 1979, updated 1988.

---

cancer, according to the National Cancer Institute and the American Cancer Society. It is recommended we consume foods containing these nutrients daily (12).

Protecting the Nutrients in Your Food

Certain vitamins are easily destroyed during food preparation and cooking, so some uncooked servings each day are recommended. A few additional guidelines can assure that you get the most from the foods you buy:

- Store fruits and vegetables in the refrigerator. Warm temperatures speed up natural enzyme processes that break down vitamins once food is harvested.
- Keep fruits and vegetables from being exposed to the air and wrap cut surfaces before storing to preserve vitamin C.
- Slice fruits and vegetables as close to cooking or serving time as possible. Leaving broccoli chopped and sitting on the cutting board for 15 minutes results in large amounts of vitamin C lost, for example.

- Boiling vegetables results in loss of water-soluble nutrients into the water. This cooking water can be refrigerated for later use in soups and sauces, but steaming vegetables avoids much of this loss. If you do boil vegetables, cut them in large rather than small pieces. Boil potatoes in their skins.
- Buy fresh and frozen fruits and vegetables rather than canned to obtain more vitamins B_6, pantothenic acid, and folacin.
- Vitamin A is destroyed by air and light; riboflavin is destroyed by light. Buy milk in cartons rather than glass bottles if the grocery store dairy case is exposed to light.

MINERALS

Minerals are as basic as chemicals get; they are atoms of inorganic elements, indestructible, derived from the earth's crust, absorbed through plant roots, incorporated into plant tissue, and ultimately into the structure of our own bones and teeth. They are integral parts of the regulatory mechanisms and enzyme systems in the body, as well. Minerals help to regulate fluid balance, transport substances throughout the body, allow muscles to contract, and nerves to transmit signals, and perform countless other functions.

Like vitamins, minerals can perform their functions repeatedly and at lightning speed. For example, one crucial zinc atom set in the center of a particular enzyme in the lungs comes into contact with 600,000 of its target molecules, carbonic acid, each second. As a result, carbonic acid is broken apart into water and carbon dioxide, and the carbon dioxide is excreted in our breath. To perform this and numerous other tasks, only a few milligrams of zinc are needed in the diet each day, a speck, barely visible to the eye but wondrously hardworking and essential to life.

Iron
In the United States, low intakes of calcium and iron are of concern among certain population groups (13). Inadequate iron intake is the most common nutritional deficiency among women and young children. Without iron, oxygen cannot be transported and anemia results, causing fatigue and susceptibility to infection. Red meats, organ meats, legumes, dark green leafy vegetables, and breads and grains are good sources of iron. Although many people need to cut back on fatty meats, here is a situation in which frequent inclusion of lean red meats in the diet is beneficial.

(continued on p. 127)

Table 5.2 About Minerals

Mineral	Function	Best Sources	Comments
Calcium	Muscle action, blood clotting, bones and teeth	Milk, cheese, greens, canned fish (with bones)	Deficiency common in women
Phosphorus	Bones and teeth, DNA, enzyme reactions	Protein foods, processed foods, soft drinks	Excess contributes to poor bone health
Magnesium	Muscle action, heartbeat, enzyme reactions	Whole grains, blackstrap molasses	Found in hard water; mild deficiency may be common in highly processed diets
Sodium	Acid-base balance, fluid balance, muscle action, nerve transmission	Salt, snack foods, salt-cured meats, food additives, pickled foods, processed foods	Excess intake linked to salt-sensitive hypertension
Potassium	Acid-base balance, heartbeat, enzyme reactions	Fruits, potatoes, blackstrap molasses	Mild deficiency may contribute to hypertension
Iron	Oxygen transportation in red blood cells	Red meats, grains, liver, prunes, dark green leafy vegetables	Deficiency common in children and women; causes anemia
Zinc	Role in numerous enzyme reactions	Seafood, meat, whole grains (not enriched), eggs, nuts	Excessive amounts impair copper and iron absorption
Iodine	Component of thyroid hormone	Iodized salt, seafood	
Chromium	Aids action of insulin	Whole grains, blackstrap molasses, mushrooms, wheat germ	Deficiency may contribute to adult-onset diabetes
Selenium	Component of antioxidant enzymes	Grains, meat, milk products	Amount in food dependent on selenium in soil. Narrow range between safe and toxic amount

Minerals help to regulate fluid balance, transport substances around the body, allow muscles to contract, and nerves to transmit signals. Like vitamins, they are spread through different food groups so variety is essential to ensure adequacy of intake.

Did You Know That . . .

Six to 12 iron tablets can kill a young person, and among children, iron poisoning deaths are second only to poisonings from aspirin overdose.

Do You Get Enough Iron?*

Food	Serving size	Iron (mg per serving)
beef liver	3 oz	4.0
oysters	4	3.6
chicken liver	3 oz	3.2
pork roast	3 oz	3.2
roast beef	3 oz	3.1
leg of lamb	3 oz	1.9
fillet of sole	3 oz	1.4
chicken breast	1	1.3
egg	1	1.3
navy beans, cooked	1 cup	5.0
black-eyed peas, cooked	1 cup	4.8
green peas	1 cup	2.9
spinach, cooked	1/2 cup	2.1
potato, baked	1	1.1
kale, cooked	1/2 cup	.9
collard greens, cooked	1/2 cup	.8
broccoli, cooked	1/2 cup	.6
40% bran flakes	1 cup	12.0
whole wheat or enriched bread	1 slice	1.5
rice	1/2 cup	.5
macaroni, enriched	1/2 cup	.6
oatmeal	1/2 cup	.7
prune juice	1 cup	10.5
prunes, cooked	1/2 cup	2.1
strawberries	1 cup	1.5
blackstrap molasses	1 tablespoon	3.2

*RDA for females age 15–50: 15 mg, females age 51 and older: 10 mg
RDA for males age 15–18: 12 mg, males age 19 and older: 10 mg

Meeting a woman's iron need:

4 slices whole wheat bread	6.0
1/2 cup beans	2.5
lean beef, 3 oz	3.1
baked potato	1.1
strawberries, 1 cup	1.5
1/2 cup oatmeal	.7
1/2 cup broccoli	.6
	15.5 mg

Source: U.S. Department of Agriculture, Handbook No. 456.

Hematocrits and hemoglobin tests measure the iron in blood and are available through health clinics and physician's offices. If iron in the blood is low, several dietary steps can be taken. The iron in meat (heme iron) is in a more absorbable form than the iron in legumes, grains, and vegetables (nonheme iron), so more of it is picked up from the digestive tract and carried into the blood. In addition, foods with vitamin C eaten with foods rich in iron aid the absorption of iron. This vitamin C-plus-iron combination is especially important for vegetarians who consume the less absorbable nonheme iron in plant foods. Examples of iron-vitamin C combinations are bean dishes served with broccoli or cabbage coleslaw, burritos with tomato slices, oatmeal with a slice of cantaloupe, and a peanut butter sandwich with orange juice. Using cast-iron cookware also adds iron to the diet.

Calcium

A second mineral of particular concern to women is calcium, a major mineral in bones. A condition called osteoporosis, in which bones become increasingly porous and brittle, affects many older women in this country. The factors involved in its onset include a low calcium intake, changes in female sex hormones after menopause, a sedentary life-style, too much phosphorus or protein in the diet, cigarette smoking, heredity, and a small bone structure.

Studies show nearly one-third of the women in the United States consume only half the calcium they need (13). Habits that can be started early in life to develop strong bones and minimize risk of osteoporosis in later years include consuming adequate calcium (800 to 1200 milligrams daily), avoiding too many protein foods and high phosphorus foods (meat, soft drinks, processed foods), not smoking, and taking part in regular, weight-bearing physical activity (such as walking, jogging, cycling). It appears particularly important to have adequate dietary calcium up to the age of 24, when bone growth stops (14). Bone density continues to increase for many years after this, however, and adequate calcium intake remains important throughout life.

Sodium

Sodium receives much attention in the media for its role in hypertension. Although too much sodium appears to be a problem for a segment of the population, it is an essential nutrient that is obtained through the diet. Sodium is needed for nerve signals, muscle contraction and relaxation, and acid-base balance. It is one of the main factors in the body's regulation of fluid balance via control of urine production and the thirst mechanism.

Table 5.3 Calcium in Foods

		Mg Per Serving
whole milk	1 cup	290
skim milk	1 cup	302
yogurt	1 cup	270
cheddar cheese	1 ounce	213
cottage cheese	¹/₂ cup	100
ice cream	1 cup	194
canned salmon	3.5 ounces	225
sardines	3 ounces	375
tofu	2 in. × 1 in. piece	154
spinach, cooked	¹/₂ cup	116
broccoli, cooked	¹/₂ cup	68
okra, cooked	¹/₂ cup	147
lentils	¹/₂ cup	25
lima beans	¹/₂ cup	40
orange	1	70
cornbread	2 in. square	133
blackstrap molasses	1 tbs	137
raisins	3 tbs	54

RDA for males and females age 15–24: 1200 mg, age 25 and older: 800 mg

Source: U.S. Department of Agriculture, Handbook No. 456.

Inadequate calcium intake is a particular concern among women in the United States, one-third of whom consume half the recommended daily amount according to recent studies. While milk and dairy products are perhaps the best-known source of this essential mineral, there are many others, some of which are shown above.

About 30 percent of adults in the United States have hypertension, or chronic high blood pressure, which increases risk of heart disease, kidney disease, and stroke (15). Genetics, stress, smoking, and overweight are major predisposing factors. For approximately one-third to one-half of hypertensives, too much sodium is involved (16). Other minerals are implicated in hypertension as well, particularly low calcium and potassium intakes, but the association with sodium remains the strongest. The Dietary Guidelines for Americans recommend we "avoid too much sodium" and the National Research Council states salt should be limited to 6 grams a day (1 teaspoon). Americans typically take in 2 to 3 teaspoons a day (17).

Enough sodium to support health occurs naturally in foods. In the American diet, large amounts of sodium come from table salt (which is 40 percent sodium), processed and convenience foods, canned foods, luncheon meats, food additives such as sodium nitrite and monosodium glutamate, condiments such as catsup, steak sauce, soy sauce, and pickles, baking mixes which

(continued on p. 131)

A ccording to the Center for Science in the Public Interest, the average sodium content in processed foods has declined by about 2 percent a year since 1984. Frozen dinners and canned soups still provide 75 percent of the sodium in the American diet.

If you are one of the many Americans contributing to the $318 million spent annually on calcium supplements in an effort to build up stores of the mineral, there's something you should know. The calcium in a number of these tablets never makes it to your bones; most of it goes straight through the digestive tract without being absorbed. Ironically, supplements that contain the greatest concentrations of calcium are among the ones the body cannot make use of.

Not All Calcium Pills Provide Calcium

These pills are composed of calcium carbonate, a compound that contains more calcium by weight than any other supplement on the market. Acid in the stomach normally breaks up calcium carbonate into tiny pieces that can easily be dissolved and then absorbed into the bloodstream. But when manufacturers compress larger and larger amounts of calcium into smaller and smaller pills, it becomes more difficult for stomach acid to break them up. Tablets that are touted as "starch-free" can also hamper the stomach's ability to perform its job. (Starch is a disintegrating agent that helps calcium pills break apart. Minute amounts are used in many formulations.)

To be sure, most of the major suppliers of supplements made of calcium carbonate, such as OS-Cal, Caltrate-D, and Tums, manufacture pills that are easily dissolvable, says Ralph Shangraw, PhD, a University of Maryland School of Pharmacy researcher who has studied the calcium supplements on the market to determine how absorbable they are. The products that fail to dissolve properly are private brand supplements made by small companies and marketed under such names as Medicine Shoppe Cal.-D, General Nutrition Center Calcium-D 600, and Ames Calcium-D 600. The manufacturers of these pills have not been deliberately attempting to defraud the public; it's simply that many small companies can't afford to formulate and test their products properly.

The firms whose supplements have been found to be of poor quality are working to reformulate them. In the meantime, a pharmacist may be of help to you in weeding out poor-quality supplements. If that is not possible, Dr. Shangraw recommends a simple, do-it-yourself test. Drop a single calcium-carbonate tablet into six ounces of vinegar, which mimics the acid environment of the stomach, stirring occasionally. After 30 minutes, a high-quality formulation should break up and be 75 percent dissolved, according to the United States Pharmacopeia, a nonprofit group that sets voluntary standards for drugs. Lack of disintegration is a clear indication of a calcium-carbonate product with a poor formulation.

Once you find a dissolvable calcium-carbonate supplement, you can enhance its absorption by following two simple guidelines. First, drink at least six to eight ounces of water or fluid with the tablet to help break it down. And second, take the tablet at mealtime, because the presence of food in the stomach maximizes acid secretion and thereby helps dissolve it. Unfortunately, however, swallowing calcium supplements with meals may interfere with the absorption of iron.

Certainly, taking a calcium supplement is one approach. However, eating such foods as dairy products, salmon, and leafy green vegetables rather than swallowing a pill is preferable—especially because you get added nutrients with food.

Source: *Tufts University Diet & Nutrition Letter,* Vol. 6, No. 2, April 1988.

Table 5.4 Sample Food Selections to Meet Daily Calcium Need for Adults Under Age 25

With Milk Products:

2 cups skim milk	604
2 ounces cheddar cheese	426
1 orange	70
1/2 cup broccoli	68
	1168 mg

Without Milk Products:

2 pieces tofu	308
1 cup spinach	232
3.5 oz canned salmon	225
1 orange	70
1 cup lima beans	80
2 pieces cornbread	266
	1181 mg

Source: *Environmental Nutrition,* April 1988.

It is particularly important for both men and women to have adequate dietary calcium up to age 24 when bone growth stops. The quantity needed can be obtained either with or without milk products, although diets without milk products require more attention to good calcium sources.

FIGURE 5.1
Sources of Dietary Sodium

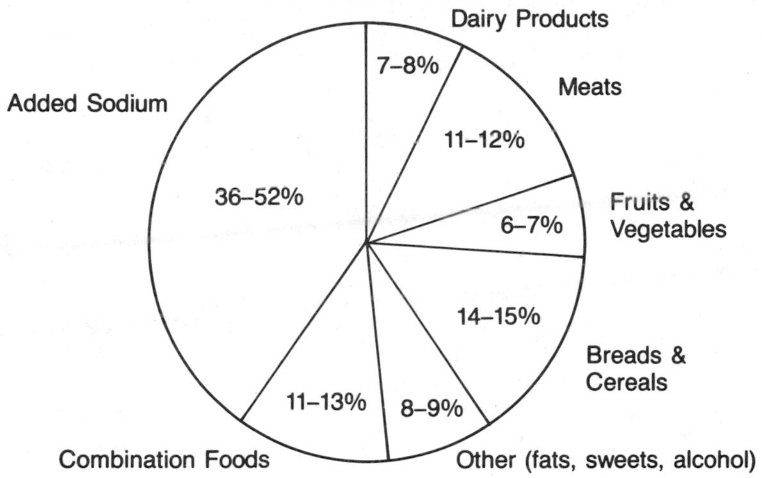

Source: *Environmental Nutrition,* April 1988.

The intake of sodium recommended by The Food and Nutrition Board of the National Academy of Sciences ranges from 1,100 to 3,500 milligrams per day, but most Americans consume two to three times that amount. From one-third to one-half of this intake comes from salt added to processed foods.

Did You Know That . . .

Saltwater fish generally contain no more sodium than freshwater fish because the internal regulatory system in saltwater fish prevents the absorption of sodium from the ocean.

contain baking soda, luncheon meats, and fast foods. A typical fast-food cheeseburger provides four times the sodium needed for an entire day. A serving of canned soup provides over twice the daily need. Eating most foods close to their natural state and limiting convenience food items and salt sprinkled on food can result in significant reductions in sodium intake.

SUMMARY

Although vitamins, minerals, and water do not provide energy in the sense of fuel the body can use, they are essential to feeling energetic, staying healthy, and preventing disease. Vitamins and minerals are spread throughout the different food groups, so variety in choices is important to ensure adequacy of these nutrients. Unprocessed foods generally contain more vitamins and minerals than processed foods, so we should consume most

FIGURE 5.2
Estimating the Sodium in Your Diet

Take a look at how the foods you eat and the way you prepare and serve them affect the amount of sodium in your diet.

How Often Do You:	Less Than Once a Week	1 or 2 Times a Week	3 to 5 Times a Week	Almost Daily
1. Eat cured or processed meats such as ham, bacon, sausage, frankfurters, and other luncheon meats?	☐	☐	☐	☐
2. Choose canned vegetables or frozen vegetables with sauce?	☐	☐	☐	☐
3. Use commercially prepared meals, main dishes, or canned or dehydrated soups?	☐	☐	☐	☐
4. Eat cheese?	☐	☐	☐	☐
5. Eat salted nuts, popcorn, pretzels, corn chips, potato chips?	☐	☐	☐	☐
6. Add salt to cooking water for vegetables, rice, or pasta?	☐	☐	☐	☐
7. Add salt, seasoning mixes, salad dressings, or condiments such as soy sauce, steak sauce, catsup, and mustard to foods during preparation or at the table?	☐	☐	☐	☐
8. Salt your food before tasting it?	☐	☐	☐	☐

How Did You Do?
The more checks you have in the last two columns, the higher your diet is likely to be in sodium. However, not all of the items listed contribute the same amount of sodium. For example, many natural cheeses are relatively low in sodium. Most processed cheeses and cottage cheese are higher.

To cut back on sodium, you can start by having some items less often, particularly those you checked as "3 to 5 times a week" or more. This does not mean eliminating foods from your diet. You can moderate your sodium intake by choosing lower sodium foods from each food group more often and by balancing high-sodium foods with low-sodium ones. For example, if you serve ham for dinner, plan to serve it with fresh or plain frozen vegetables cooked without added salt.

Source: U.S Department of Agriculture *Home and Garden Bulletin* No. 232–6, April 1986.

foods in their basic, untampered-with state. This same advice has been given, in various guises, in previous chapters. Whether the diet needs more variety; less fat, sugar, or sodium; more fiber, calcium, or complex carbohydrates; or more foods protective against cancer, the types of foods recommended to achieve a healthy balance remain consistent: whole grains, cereals and breads, legumes, fruits, vegetables, lean meats, fish, poultry, and low-fat milk products. 〽

Making Choices

MANY FACTORS BEYOND the nutrient content of foods affect health. Not just what is eaten, but when and how often impacts on nutritional state, energy level, and mood. One's emotional state can also impact on food choices. People may choose comfort foods when sad, depressed, or lonely. How one thinks about food can be involved, too; severe anxiety about food and calories among a high percentage of teenage and college-age women has been correlated with poor nutrient intakes.

DIET AND WELL-BEING

Mental state can affect physiological processes in the body. When feeling hurried, under stress, or upset, blood supply to the digestive tract can be restricted and gastric acid secretion in the stomach can increase. Eating at such a time might result in indigestion or heartburn. Mood changes caused by diet can also occur. For example, the depression often seen in dieters is suspected of being caused by reduced levels of **serotonin**, a natural tranquilizing hormone produced in the brain only when adequate carbohydrate is present (1). Drinking over 5 cups of coffee a day can result in anxiety, irritability, headaches, insomnia and nervousness, a condition termed **caffeinism** (2). Nutrients and other food components are being discovered to affect brain function and moods in ways we are just starting to understand.

We are the best judges of how all these factors fit into our total nutritional picture. By beginning to pay attention to how our food choices affect us and how our feelings affect our food choices, we can make positive changes in our diet. A good place to start is by looking at our meal patterns.

Serotonin: A neurotransmitter in the brain formed from the amino acid tryptophan that may have a role in modulating sleep and pain.

Caffeinism: A response to an overdose of caffeine that resembles an anxiety attack with dizziness, agitation, sleep difficulties, restlessness, and headache.

133

Pizza for Breakfast?

Are three square meals a day really necessary? What makes a good meal? Fortunately, there are no hard and fast rules. What is important is consuming the foods we need and enjoy during the day in a way that suits us.

It is true, however, that some eating patterns are more likely to result in a well-nourished state than others. A food life-style that involves grabbing quick meals and snacks on the run is generally associated with a less nutritious diet than one planned around regular mealtimes (3). There is no reason, however, why snacking shouldn't fit into the day's pattern if wise choices are made. Breakfast may be important to fuel the morning's activities, but breakfast doesn't have to be limited to eggs or cereal; some people prefer leftover pizza. Either choice provides adequate nutrition. Similarly, a bowl of cereal with milk and fruit on top can pass for dinner, assuming foods earlier in the day provided enough other nutrients to meet one's needs.

In general, approaches to meals and snacking differ and no right way applies to everyone. Some people prefer three meals a day, others two, and still others several small meals or snacks. Busy students and harried professionals can fall into a pattern where they typically go for long periods without eating (routinely skipping lunch, for example) and don't realize the toll it takes on their energy level until they try a more optimal pattern. In assessing our own meal patterns, we should consider how long we go between eating. Is it more than 4 or 5 hours? If so, feelings of tiredness and irritability would be understandable and the solution is obvious. If allowing time for meals is difficult, we should plan to pack foods, carry them in our cars, or store them in our desk.

Physical Activity

It is best to be physically active for the enjoyment and energy it brings. We should realize, however, that physical activity, or the lack of it, greatly influences our nutritional state. Exercise improves the circulatory system which brings nutrients to the cells, and carries waste away from them. Perspiration during exercise allows excretion of waste products. Regular exercise helps control imbalances in cholesterol and is an important adjunct to a low-fat diet for those with elevated cholesterol. Done outdoors, synthesis of vitamin D occurs as the sun's rays strike our skin. Exercise also improves the health of bones. The pressure put on bones during a simple physical activity such as walking stimulates them to draw calcium from the blood and place it

(continued on p. 137)

The custom of eating a meal at the start of the day is observed in cultures all over the world. Does this make breakfast man's most important meal? Perhaps. Research, for instance, shows that eating breakfast improves intellectual performance and the ability to concentrate and solve problems at the same time as it increases the nutrient content of a person's diet. On the flip side, skipping breakfast has been proven to cause fatigue, decrease the body's metabolic rate, increase snacking during the day and lead to weight gain.

The A.M. Meal Makes a Difference

Most research on the importance of breakfast has been done with children. Studies show that test scores improve when children are given a morning meal. Not that cereal, milk and juice make kids smarter, but their attention span is increased making it possible for more learning to take place.

Breakfast eaters (both children and adults) consume more essential nutrients like calcium, fiber and vitamins C, B-1 and B-2 than do breakfast skippers. Generally speaking, better nutrition means better resistance to infection.

Stretching that point even further, results of a University of California study showed that breakfast eaters actually lived longer than breakfast skippers. Of course, other factors could be responsible for the findings. For example, people who eat breakfast may also exercise more, and the activity could be the factor responsible for their longevity. Still, the California finding is a provocative one.

Probably the most compelling argument in support of a morning repast is its role in weight management. When a person gets up in the morning with an empty stomach, blood sugar is literally at a "fasting" or very low level. Eating shortly after rising causes the body's furnace to heat up as it burns off the calories of that first meal. Called the "thermic effect of food," it increases after each meal throughout the day. Skipping breakfast, on the other hand, keeps the furnace cold longer and ultimately burns fewer calories.

People who don't eat breakfast have metabolic rates four to five percent below normal, according to Wayne Calloway, M.D. of George Washington University, Washington D.C. As a result of this metabolic slump, a breakfast skipper could expect to gain one pound every seven weeks (about 8 pounds per year)—even if his calorie intake remained the same.

Clearly, breakfast is a good idea. To those who say they can't eat in the morning, Dr. Calloway replies, "Nonsense." Eating is an environmental response, he says. And breakfast skippers must condition themselves to eat in the morning by eating lighter and earlier the night before. Even a confirmed breakfast skipper will soon find himself waking up hungry, says Calloway.

But what constitutes a good morning meal? The answer is not as pat as the bacon-and-eggs menu at the local coffee shop would suggest. The choices for breakfast are unlimited. Here are a few quick a.m. menu options:

Leftover Pudding

Combine tonight's leftover rice, macaroni, stale bread, kasha or couscous with lowfat milk, chopped fruit, beaten egg white and the sweetener and seasonings of your choice. Bake until set. Refrigerate overnight and scoop up a quick dish in the morning.

Sunrise Stuffed Potatoes

Bake a potato in the microwave oven. Then split it and fill with some leftovers in the fridge—chili, spaghetti sauce, low-fat cheese, stew, pea soup—whatever is appealing—then reheat.

Layered Breakfast 'Shortcakes'

Start with a frozen waffle or pancake. Drop it in the toaster. Then spread on a layer of peanut butter, warm applesauce or other fruit puree, vanilla yogurt or cinnamon-sprinkled cottage cheese. Now top it off with a teaspoon of chopped nuts, juice-packed canned fruit or nugget-type cereal.

Breakfast Pizzas

For something really different, try the a.m. version of pizza. Individual pizzas are easy to make with English muffins or bagels topped with part skim mozzarella cheese and ham slices or Canadian bacon (both are low-fat). Experienced breakfast eaters may even want to add a spicy tomato sauce (left over or from a jar); but it may be too much for beginners.

Cereal Sundaes

To make standard breakfast cereals more exciting, make up zip-lock bags full of add-ins like chopped dried apricots, banana chips, almonds, toasted wheat germ and raisins. Mix and match these "sundae toppings" to create a different cereal every morning. They're just as good with hot cereals as they are with cold.

High Fiber Yogurt

For people with little time in the morning to sit down for breakfast, take a carton of plain, vanilla or lemon yogurt and stir a crunchy, high-fiber cereal right into the yogurt carton. It's satisfying, nutritious and it's portable.

—*Robyn Flipse, M.S., R.D.*

Source: *Environmental Nutrition,* Vol. 12, No. 9, September 1989, p. 2.

within their mineral matrix, making them stronger. **Aerobic exercise** reduces excess stores of body fat and most types of exercise stimulate the building of new muscle. Physical activity keeps the metabolic rate high, greatly aiding long-term weight management. Being active thus goes hand in hand with many dietary factors to provide an optimal state of nutrition, body composition, and overall health.

Ethics, Values, and Beliefs

For many, food choices involve more than personal taste or health considerations. As discussed in chapter 4, some people are choosing to eat less meat and more plant foods as a personal response to world hunger and environmental issues. Others choose to buy or raise food grown without pesticides and chemical fertilizers in an effort to promote a healthy ecology of the land and water. Still others choose a completely vegetarian diet based on moral or spiritual considerations. Rather than unpleasant restrictions, these choices can be seen as an individual's way of living his or her philosophy of life and putting spiritual values into daily action. And as such, these commitments add depth to our culture just as the putting into practice of ethical precepts and values adds depth to our individual natures (see the Resources section at the end of this book for further readings on world hunger, agricultural, and environmental issues).

FOOD CONSUMERISM

As buyers in the food and nutrition marketplace, we are faced with a bewildering array of products, information, and claims about everything from food additives to nutritional supplements to fast foods. Here, a little knowledge and a healthy dose of skepticism can go a long way.

The Advertising Shuffle

A portion of every dollar we spend on food is used by manufacturers to promote their products via commercials, catchy packaging, magazine and billboard ads, in-store displays, and special promotions to supermarket chain buyers. The law of the marketplace is to increase sales. Products from candy bars to breakfast cereals to natural potato chips are touted as nutritious, not because food manufacturers are necessarily concerned about our health, but because they know nutrition is a selling point that helps their product move off the shelf and into the grocery cart. The dilemma for consumers lies in determining which products

Aerobic exercise: Exercise in which the body is able to meet the muscles' increased demand for oxygen continuously during increased activity. Aerobic means "requiring air to live."

(continued on p. 140)

Coffee: Benign Beverage or Dangerous Drink?

Whether it's regular or decaf, *café au lait* or espresso, coffee is one of the world's most popular beverages. It may also be the most controversial.

Seldom has a substance been the subject of so many conflicting studies of its health effects. To date, coffee has been implicated in such "public enemy" diseases, as heart disease and cancer. Yet completely conclusive evidence to support the accusations is lacking. In fact, the more studies that are completed, the more coffee seems to be exonerated. Is coffee dangerous, or is it a benign beverage?

Heart Disease: The Pulse of the Issue. Coffee was first linked to heart disease in the early 1970's when reports claimed that people who consumed one to five, and six or more cups of coffee per day increased by 50% and 120%, respectively, their risk of heart attack.(1)

This finding led to a multitude of studies of the coffee-heart relationship. The largest, the Framingham Heart Study, tracked 5,000 people over 40 years. Coffee consumption was evaluated as a part of the study. It concluded that coffee was not linked to higher incidences of death from heart disease, even among people with high blood pressure.

Other studies have tended to contradict one another. In 1985, a Stanford University study showed middle-aged men more likely to have high blood cholesterol when they drank more than 2½ to 3 cups of coffee per day. A study completed in 1987 at the University of Pittsburgh, however, showed the opposite to be true: that coffee drinkers did not have dangerously high levels of blood cholesterol—and, in fact, women coffee drinkers tended to have lower blood triglyceride levels than non-coffee drinkers.(2) Because of the inconsistencies of these findings, researchers haven't been able to get to the "heart" of the issue. Finally, in the summer of 1988, the U.S. Surgeon General reported that the evidence of a relationship between coffee drinking and coronary heart disease was too weak to recommend that Americans decrease their coffee consumption.

The Coffee-Cancer Connection. Dozens of studies have tried to uncover a link between coffee and different types of cancer. One such study at Harvard University caused a stir when it claimed coffee consumption to be linked to pancreatic cancer.(3) But the study was highly criticized, and follow-up studies by other scientists failed to support its conclusion.

Other studies of bladder, breast and ovarian cancers, have not found a concrete link with coffee consumption. To cap it off, the American Cancer Society issued a statement in 1984 specifying that coffee does not increase risk of cancer.

Fibrocystic Breast Disease. Yet another health concern in which coffee is implicated is fibrocystic breast disease, a condition of painful benign lumps in breast tissue. In 1979, reports linked reduced symptoms of fibrocystic breast disease in women who cut methylxanthines (stimulants, of which caffeine is one) from their diets. Since then, several conflicting studies have been published.

A study published in the *Journal of the National Cancer Institute* in 1984 found a positive association between methylxanthine consumption including caffeine, and fibrocystic breast disease.(4) But another large study published in the *American Journal of Epidemiology* in 1986 concluded there was no association between methylxanthine consumption and risk of fibrocystic breast disease.(5) The jury is still out.

Birth Defects. Although no human studies support the claim that high coffee intake can cause birth defects, animal studies have shown an increased incidence of birth defects in pregnant rats fed large doses of caffeine directly into their stomachs.

On the other hand, a recent study conducted by the Food and Drug Administration, in which caffeine was fed to pregnant rats in their drinking water, concluded that caffeine was not related to birth defects.

Caffeine does, however, cross the placenta, and fetuses are not able to metabolize. Caffeine may linger in fetal tissue for three to four days following consumption. As a precautionary measure, the FDA recommends that women not drink more than two or three cups of coffee per day during pregnancy.

Though there doesn't appear to be a relationship between coffee and birth defects, a recent study offers women new cause for concern. (See *EN* February 1989.) Researchers found that women who consumed more caffeine than is found in a single cup of coffee experienced a decline in fertility and were only half as likely to become pregnant during any given month as women who consumed less caffeine.

Digestive Disorders. Caffeine promotes heartburn by lessening the pressure in the lower part of the esophagus (esophageal sphincter). Coffee (not caffeine, *per se*) also stimulates gastric acid secretion. For this reason, people with peptic ulcer disease should avoid coffee—even decaffeinated blends.

Other Health Issues. Caffeine is indisputably a mild stimulant of the central nervous system. Depending on how sensitive a person is, it can cause "jitters," tremors, heart palpitations, insomnia and other signs of agitation.

Caffeine is also a mild diuretic. There is however, a tolerance effect—the more coffee a person drinks on a regular basis, the less likely he is to be bothered by the diuretic effect. Actually, this may tell us something more significant. The tolerance developed by chronic coffee drinking may be one reason why results of caffeine and coffee studies exhibit such wide discrepancies.

For example, an article in the *Annals of Internal Medicine* in 1983, suggested that although coffee influences blood pressure, blood sugar (in diabetics), plasma catecholamine (a type of neurotransmitter) levels, serum cholesterol levels and urine production, *chronic* coffee consumption seems to cause none, or less of these effects.

What to Do. The overwhelming majority of coffee and health research seems to suggest casting aside suspicions of coffee as an evil beverage. New studies suggest instead that moderate coffee drinkers (people who drink two to three 5 or 6-ounce cups a day) may have little cause for worry. As in so many nutrition-related questions, moderation seems to be the key.

—*Linda Weinberg, R.D.*

1. *The New England Journal of Medicine*, pp. 63–67, July 12, 1973.
2. *Athersclerosis*, pp. 97–103, October 1987.
3. *The New England Journal of Medicine*, pp. 630–633, March 12, 1981.
4. *Journal of the National Cancer Institute*, pp. 1015–1019, May, 1984.
5. *American Journal of Epidemiology*, pp. 603–611, October, 1986.

Source: *Environmental Nutrition*, Vol. 12, No. 8, August 1989.

Caffeine Contents of Coffee and Other Products

If avoiding caffeine is the main concern, note that coffee is not the only caffeine containing product people consume. Since 1985, soft drinks have surpassed coffee as the largest source of caffeine in American diets. Other sources of caffeine are listed below.

Product	Amount	Caffeine (milligrams)
Coffee, brewed	10 ounce mug	230
Dexatrim	1 capsule	200
Coffee, brewed	5 ounce cup	115
Aqua-ban	1 tablet	100
NoDoz	1 tablet	100
Coffee, instant	5 ounce cup	80
Jolt	12 ounce can	72
Excedrin	1 capsule	65
Mountain Dew	12 ounce can	54
Mello Yello	12 ounce can	53
Tea, brewed	5 ounce cup	50
Coke	12 ounce can	46
Pepsi	12 ounce can	39
Anacin	1 tablet	32
Tea, instant	5 ounce cup	30
Coffee, decaffeinated, brewed	5 ounce cup	3
Coffee, decaffeinated, instant	5 ounce cup	2

Sources of information: National Coffee Association, New York, New York; National Soft Drink Association, Washington, D.C.; Physicians Desk Reference for OTC Drugs, 1988.

Lo-Cal

Lite

100% Natural

Organic
Low Cholesterol
Pure

Wholesome

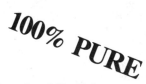

100% PURE

No Artificial
Ingredients

Whole Grains

are as nutritious as the manufacturer claims. Is a potato chip with the skin left on and containing no preservatives really more nutritious than a standard potato chip, when both are loaded with fat and salt?

Deciphering Food Labels

How can we tell whether a food is what the advertiser claims it is? Since the aim of food advertising is to sell food, advertisers play to our basic needs and desires: to be slim, beautiful, handsome, sexy, healthy, and to have a particular social status—a gourmet, a jet-setter, in touch with nature, a good parent, etc. Label buzzwords match the current interests and concerns of the public, so we now see everywhere the terms "lite," "lo-cal," "all natural," "high energy," "nutritious," "contains no preservatives," "organic," and "wholesome." Of these terms, only "lo-cal" has a legally defined meaning. The others are no guarantee the product is what we think it is.

Look at advertisements and package claims with a skeptical eye and examine the ingredients list on the package. They are listed in order of predominance by weight, so the ingredient present in the highest amount is listed first. For example, a breakfast cereal that lists sugar first, contains more of it than any other ingredient and is probably not a nutritious product no matter how many vitamins have been added. If sugar or fat is the first or second ingredient, or different types of sugar or fat are listed two or three times, the product is going to be high in these substances.

Try to determine which ingredients provide the calories. Do they come from refined flour or whole grain flour? From saturated, monounsaturated, or polyunsaturated fat? From sugar or from complex carbohydrate?

Examine the nutrition label on the package, required of any product that makes a nutritional claim. Here you will find the serving size, the calories, protein, fat, carbohydrate, and sodium in a serving, and the percent of the U.S. Recommended Daily Allowances for protein, vitamins, and minerals each serving provides. The U.S. RDAs are a variation of the RDAs, which have several age and sex categories. To avoid labeling confusion, the U.S. RDA is defined as the highest value given for a nutrient on the RDA tables (excluding children under the age of 4 and pregnant and lactating women). This is generally the RDA for adult men. Some labels also provide a breakdown of the saturated fat, unsaturated fat, and cholesterol content per serving as well as the grams of sucrose, complex carbohydrates, and fiber.

(continued on p. 143)

Diet or dietetic: the food has been altered to be lower in calories, sugar, sodium, cholesterol or fat (the label must state how the food has been altered). The food is not necessarily low in calories.

Enriched: selected nutrients removed during processing have been added back in amounts close to natural levels.

Extra lean: used to describe meat products that contain no more than 5% fat.

Food Labels: What Do the Terms Mean?

Fortified: nutrients have been added that may or may not have been present in the unprocessed product or in amounts higher than those naturally present.

Imitation: the product is a substitute for and nutritionally resembles another food, such as imitation sour cream.

Lean: used to describe meat products that contain no more than 10% fat.

Leaner: used to describe meat products containing 25% less fat than the standard product.

Low calorie: the food contains no more than 40 calories per serving.

Low sodium: less than 140 mg sodium per serving.

Reduced calorie: the food is at least one-third lower in calories than the comparable food it resembles.

Reduced sodium: sodium content is 25% lower than the original food or product.

Sodium-free: less than 5 mg sodium per serving.

Substitute: the product is a substitute for another food but is nutritionally inferior.

Sugar-free or sugarless: the food contains no table sugar (sucrose) but can contain other caloric sweeteners such as corn syrup, fructose, sorbitol or honey.

Unsalted: processed with no additional salt, although some sodium may be present naturally in the food.

Terms with no legal definition

Light and lite: the food could be lighter in sodium, calories, sugar, color, taste, or texture.

Natural

Organic

Organically grown (except in the few states that legally define this term)

FIGURE 6.1
Food Label

Lean Cuisine®
Single Serving

Stouffer's

Cheese Cannelloni
with Tomato Sauce

NUTRITIONAL FACTS

	Cheese Cannelloni	Daily dietary guidelines for healthy adults†
CHOLESTEROL	35 mg	Less than 300 mg
SODIUM	910 mg	Less than 3000 mg
FAT	90 cal	Less than 420 calories from fat*

*Based on average calorie-controlled intake of 1400 calories

†These dietary guidelines are based on published daily dietary recommendations from leading health organizations.

© Stouffer Foods Corporation

INFORMATION PANEL

NUTRITION INFORMATION	PER SERVING	NUTRITION INFORMATION	PER SERVING
SERVING SIZE	9⅛ OZ.	FAT	10g
SERVINGS PER CONTAINER	1	POLYUNSATURATED FAT	1g
CALORIES	260	SATURATED FAT	5g
PROTEIN	21g	CHOLESTEROL	35mg
CARBOHYDRATE	22g	SODIUM	910mg

PERCENTAGE OF U.S. RECOMMENDED DAILY ALLOWANCE (U.S. RDA)

PROTEIN	30	RIBOFLAVIN	15
VITAMIN A	15	NIACIN	6
VITAMIN C	10	CALCIUM	30
THIAMINE	8	IRON	4

INGREDIENTS: WATER, COOKED MACARONI PRODUCT, DRY CURD COTTAGE CHEESE, RICOTTA CHEESE, TOMATO PUREE, TOMATOES WITH PUREE, LOW-MOISTURE PART-SKIM MOZZARELLA CHEESE, TOMATOES, PARMESAN CHEESE, CARROTS, ONIONS, ENRICHED BLEACHED FLOUR (WHEAT FLOUR, NIACIN, REDUCED IRON, THIAMINE MONONITRATE, RIBOFLAVIN), **MODIFIED CORNSTARCH, SALT, BEEF, CORN OIL, DEHYDRATED ONIONS, MONO-SODIUM GLUTAMATE, HYDROLYZED VEGETABLE PROTEINS, XANTHAN GUM, SPICES, SUGAR, CARAMEL COLORING, DEHYDRATED GARLIC, ERYTHORBIC ACID, DRIED BEEF STOCK, SOLUBLE BAY SALT, ANTIOXIDANT** (CORN OIL, BHT, TBHQ), **NATURAL FLAVORINGS, CITRIC ACID.**

STOUFFER FOODS, SOLON, OHIO 44139

DIET EXCHANGES◊ (Per Serving)   2 Medium Fat Meat Exchanges   1 Starch Exchange   1 Vegetable Exchange

Lean Cuisine Diet Exchanges can be used with many weight control programs. Additional nutritional and exchange information available upon request.

◊Exchange calculations based on *Exchange Lists For Meal Planning©*, American Diabetes Association, Inc., The American Dietetic Association.

© Stouffer Foods Corporation

COOKING INSTRUCTIONS

■ **CONVENTIONAL OVEN**
1. Preheat oven to 375°F. Place a baking sheet on lower oven rack.
2. Place loosely covered container on middle oven rack; cook 30 minutes. Remove foil overwrap; continue cooking 10-15 minutes. <u>Carefully</u> remove from oven.

■ **MICROWAVE OVEN**
1. Remove foil overwrap; place uncovered container in oven.
2. Cook on Full power 3 minutes; rotate container ½ turn. Continue cooking on 50% power 4-5 minutes. <u>Carefully</u> remove from oven.

■ **TOASTER OVEN**
1. Preheat oven to 350°F.
2. Place loosely covered container in oven; cook 30 minutes. Remove foil overwrap; continue cooking 10-15 minutes. <u>Carefully</u> remove from oven.

Because ovens vary, these instructions are guidelines. For full enjoyment of taste and appearance, Stouffer's prefers conventional oven preparation. When time is a factor, enjoy the convenience of cooking in our microwaveable tray.

PLEASE NOTE: Our microwave instructions have been developed and tested using 600-700 watt ovens. For lower wattage ovens, additional time may be required.

MAXIMUM OVEN TEMPERATURE 375°F. DO NOT PLACE UNDER BROILER.

Please return entire Proof of Purchase Panel with correspondence relating to this product and/or health organization guidelines to: Lean Cuisine Consumer Affairs Department, Stouffer Foods, Solon, OH 44139.
Keep frozen until ready to use.

TO OPEN:
Push in pull out

Recyclable

0

13800 16636

Source: *Courtesy of Stouffer Foods,* Solon, Ohio.

The nutrition label on food packaging is a useful source of certain basic information such as serving size, the number of calories, protein, fat, carbohydrate, and sodium content in a serving, and the percent of the Recommended Daily Allowances of protein, vitamins, and minerals. Many companies, such as this one, are improving the nutrient information available on their labels so that the consumer can readily compare the amounts of cholesterol, sodium, and fat, and can also determine the number of calories from fat.

Many foods that contain refined ingredients provide adequate amounts of the nutrients listed on the label, but are low in other nutrients and fiber that are not listed. This points out a potential problem with nutrition labeling—manufacturers can take any food, add a few powdered nutrients so the label looks good and promote the food as nutritious. A food that provides vitamins and minerals can still be high in fat or sugar, or low in fiber. For example, the label on a powdered orange-flavored drink correctly states a serving contains as much vitamin C as orange juice, but vitamin C is only one of many nutrients in orange juice, which is what the orange-flavored drink is most likely replacing.

A few additional terms on labels are useful. Enriched means one or more nutrients have been added back into a product to replace selected nutrients lost during processing. These nutrients are usually replaced in amounts close to the original levels. As in the case of refined, enriched flour, however, not all nutrients lost in refining are added back in. Fortified means one or more nutrients have been added that are not naturally present in that food, or the nutrients have been added in amounts that exceed those naturally present.

Food Additives

Numerous substances are added to food products for a variety of reasons. Additives are used to thicken, emulsify (prevent ingredients from separating), leaven, add color and flavor, prevent staleness, moldiness, rancidness, discoloration, bacterial growth, and improve texture and appearance. In addition, they may be used for many other purposes. For example, some additives are necessary to preserve food products during long periods of transportation and storage.

Additives may be from natural sources, such as guar gum and agar from plants used as thickening agents. Others are synthetic copies of natural chemicals, such as ascorbic acid (vitamin C) used as an antioxidant. Still others are synthetic chemicals that have no counterpart in nature such as saccharin used in soft drinks. The most prevalent additives in our food supply are the salt, sugar, and other sweeteners added to provide flavor in numerous products. These total 93 percent of the additives we take in each year, or about 140 pounds per person. Preservatives and other chemical additives in food account for another 10 pounds (4).

The Food and Drug Administration (FDA) is responsible for regulating the use of food additives. The FDA established a Generally Recognized as Safe (GRAS) list in 1958, which includes

(continued on p. 145)

Did You Know That . . .

Annato, a yellowish-red seed extract from a small Caribbean tree, is a common food additive used to make certain cheeses yellow or orange, and many butters yellow, all of which would be a pale, creamy white without the coloring.

Did You Know That . . .

The yellow skin of chicken is due to the amount of corn in feed.

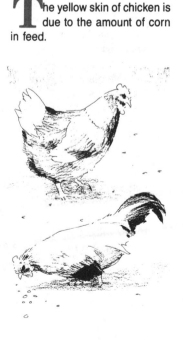

Health Foods That Aren't

Food companies strive to give us what we want, or what they think we want. And it's true that supermarkets, delis, and health-food stores now offer many excellent new products for people who watch their diet. But don't be too quick to trust those labels that promise nutritional nirvana. A food that has no cholesterol may still have lots of fat or sodium. The presence of "natural" ingredients is no guarantee of good nutrition, nor is the absence of refined sugar, preservatives, and artificial ingredients. By law, a product's ingredients are listed in descending order by weight. Thus if the whole grains you crave are near the bottom of the list, you won't be getting much of them.

Let's sample a few foods that sound promising, but often don't deliver. This doesn't mean you should rule out all of the following products—just don't be lulled into a false sense of security by a healthy-sounding name. Always read labels.

Frozen vegetarian pasta. Searching for a low-fat frozen dinner, you'll recall that pasta by itself is virtually fat-free. But prepared pasta products, even if they omit meat, often contain whole-milk cheeses, which are high in fat. A 10.5-ounce serving of one popular frozen vegetable lasagna, for instance, contains only 225 calories, but 50% of them come from the 12.5 grams of fat, which is largely saturated. The dish contains three cheeses and bread-crumb topping moistened with partially hydrogenated oils. In contrast, the percentage of fat calories in one regular meat lasagna, another frozen dinner, is only 32%.

Packaged pasta salad. These are packed like instant soups: you boil up dried pasta and dehydrated vegetables from one packet; from another, you take seasonings (including lots of sodium) to blend with oil for a dressing. But 38% of the 190 calories in a half-cup serving of one well-known brand come from eight grams of fat (seven of which you added yourself). It's better to cook your own pasta (just as quick) and add your own mix of unsalted herbs; a little Dijon mustard, chili

powder, or Worcestershire sauce combined with nonfat yogurt will perk it all up.

Bran muffins. Bakery or deli bran muffins will contain fiber if they contain bran. The question is how much. Most store-bought muffins have far more hydrogenated oils, sugar, and eggs than oat or wheat bran. Check the ingredients list: if bran is close to the bottom, you're being rooked. Look for whole-wheat flour as the main ingredient, not "wheat flour" (that is, refined white flour). If the muffin weighs heavily in your hand (some are five ounces or more) and has a sticky surface, it is likely to have as many calories and fat as any cupcake.

Carrot cake. Sure, carrots are healthful (rich in beta carotene and fiber), but carrot cakes are surprisingly rich in drawbacks. They are almost inevitably dense and moist, usually signs of a high fat content. A typical cake may contain more than a cup of oil, which has nearly 2,000 calories by itself, or about 200 calories per slice—all fat calories—before adding the other ingredients. You'll find that nearly all store-bought carrot cakes also contain a variety of sugars, refined flour, eggs, and shortening, plus cream cheese and more sugar in the frosting. In the interests of health, you'll almost always be better off with apple pie, even though it may be loaded with sugar.

Banana cake and bread. Most commercial banana cakes offer few, if any, advantages over chocolate cake. For instance, the list of ingredients in one widely sold banana cake begins with sugar, continues with partially hydrogenated vegetable shortening (partly saturated, in effect), and then flour. Only then comes the alibi for it all, bananas. Like carrot cakes, banana cakes usually get 40 to 50% of their calories from fat. You'll be better off making your own banana *bread,* which requires less fat and sugar. Store-bought banana breads, however, may be as full of fat as cakes. To avoid this, make sure flour is first on the ingredients list and shortening toward the bottom.

Frozen tofu desserts. Frozen tofu products, touted as healthful stand-ins for ice cream, are cholesterol- and lactose-free. Their calorie count and fat content, however, vary tremendously and may be higher than ice cream's. They may also be nearly tofu-free. For example, half the 230 calories in a 4-ounce serving of one well-known frozen tofu product come from sugars (high-fructose corn sweeteners, corn syrup, and honey) and the other half from fat (partially hydrogenated). Tofu ranks fifth on the ingredients list. And a chocolate (or carob) coating will add fat and calories.

Popcorn. Popcorn is a no-fat, low-calorie snack, at least when popped with little or no oil or salt (a hot-air popper requires no oil) and left unbuttered. But microwave popcorn and pre-popped corn usually contain twice as many calories as conventional popcorn, a hefty dose of salt, and more fat per ounce than most cookies. The fat comes from vegetable oils (usually hydrogenated), and sometimes from cheese as well.

Vegetarian paté. This might catch your eye as a healthy substitute for liver paté. But some vegetable patés mimic the fatty texture of traditional paté with none other than fat: for instance, one brand lists palm kernel oil (more highly saturated than animal fat) second among its ingredients, after water. Farther down the list, there's a shot of peanut oil for good measure. The predominant vegetable ingredient is potato starch.

Source: *University of California Berkeley Wellness Letter,* December 1988.

---

sugar, salt, and several hundred other substances. Additives on the GRAS list had been in the food supply for many years and were considered safe. Several substances have since been removed from the list because of safety concerns.

New additives must be tested for safety before a manufacturer can use them. Controversy exists about the accuracy and adequacy of safety tests because they are carried out by the manufacturers, who have a vested interest in declaring their products safe for consumption. In addition, short-term tests performed on laboratory animals may not be applicable to humans. Concern also exists that though an additive is determined to be safe by itself, in the presence of other chemicals or food components its safety may not be known. For example, alcoholic beverages contain additives not tested for safety in the presence of alcohol.

An important FDA law is the **Delaney Clause**, which bans from use any additive found to cause cancer in laboratory animals. This clause resulted in the banning of several food dyes and flavorings previously in use. It also resulted in a proposed FDA ban on saccharin, which was blocked by an act of Congress following intense public pressure. Saccharin remains in foods, a testament to the vigor of the dieting public, but products containing it must include a cancer warning label.

Delaney Clause: A clause in the Food, Drug, and Cosmetic Act which states that no substance known to cause cancer in animals or humans at any dose shall be added to foods.

FIGURE 6.2
Saccharin Warning Label

"Use of this product may be hazardous to your health. This product contains saccharin, which has been determined to cause cancer in laboratory animals."

Products containing saccharin are now required to have a warning label of the type shown above.

Despite questions of safety, unless one buys all food in the farm-grown state, it is impossible to avoid food additives entirely. A reasonable course is to avoid the ones with the greatest safety concerns. These additives include the synthetic food colors, which have had a poor record of safety. On labels, look for the term *artificial color* (FDC Yellow No. 5 must be named, since some people have allergic reactions to it). The National Cancer Institute recommends we avoid products containing sodium nitrite (bacon, hot dogs, and other cured meats) due to its cancer-initiation potential (5). The risks and benefits of food additives are discussed further in the box "Food Additives Offer Both Risks and Benefits" on page 147.

The Fast-Food Life-style
Although fast foods are not nutritionally ideal, they are not the complete disaster often imagined. Fast foods tend to be quite high in sodium and are often high in fat, while fruits, vegetables, and whole grains are generally underrepresented. Some fast-food hamburgers and fried chicken meals derive over half their calories from fat, and provide 10 times more sodium than we need in an entire day. On the plus side, one can obtain protein, iron, zinc, and B vitamins from hamburger patties and bean burritos; vitamin A, calcium, and riboflavin from cheese; and complex carbohydrates from buns and tortillas.

(continued on p. 149)

Food Additives Offer Both Risks and Benefits

The safety of food additives has long been a concern for Americans. Although food safety experts, government scientists and knowledgeable consumer advocates agree that most additives are safe, these groups lock horns on several issues: How should food additive laws be enforced? What risks do food additives pose to individuals compared to society? What is the scientific validity of applying animal research findings to humans?

The term food additive conjures up images of five syllable words that would stump even a chemist. In truth, most additives consumed in the U.S. are natural substances. Salt, sucrose, corn syrup, pepper, baking soda, mustard and vegetable colors—all natural—account for 98 percent, by weight, of all food additives in this country. Flavoring chemicals account for less than 1 percent by weight. Approximately 12,000 other chemicals, including pesticide and animal drug residues, are indirect or unintentional additives that inadvertently make their way into foods during food production, handling and storage.

What has raised the most concern—as well as sold newspapers and increased Nielsen ratings—are reports that certain additives cause allergic reactions in people or cancer in laboratory animals.

Without certain additives, however, bread and other baked goods would easily mold, salad oils and dressings would separate and turn rancid, salt would lump, ice cream would separate into coarse, grainy crystals, cakes wouldn't rise during baking, canned fruits and vegetables would discolor and become mushy, and foods that are now available year-round would become seasonal. Few consumers would stand for such inconvenience and poor quality.

Food Additives of Concern. Though the benefits of most food additives outweigh any possible risks, a few exist about which consumer activist groups have raised legitimate concerns. Among them are FD&C Red #3 and Yellow #5.

In September, 1989, the Public Citizen Litigation Group, a non-profit consumer advocacy group based in Washington, D.C., filed suit against the Food and Drug Administration (FDA) demanding that Red #3 be banned. The Group claims that Red #3 is an animal carcinogen. Red #3 is used primarily to color maraschino and fruit cocktail cherries and pistachio nuts.

Yellow #5 is the only color additive that is required by law to be named on product labels. It is known to cause allergic reactions in some people, especially those that are sensitive to aspirin.

Aspartame, an artificial sweetener, though deemed safe by the FDA, has been blamed for a variety of neurological and behavioral problems including headaches and dizziness. And there are concerns about using aspartame during pregnancy. It is currently found in 1,100 products in the U.S.

Residues from hormones given to livestock are indirect additives about which consumers are concerned. But, when assessing the risk they pose, it's necessary to differentiate between hormones like estrogen that are steroid-based and those like bovine somatotropine (bST) that are protein-based, according to Joseph Hotchkiss, Ph.D., Associate Professor of Food Science at Cornell University and a former FDA toxicologist.

Illegal use and overdosages of steroid-based hormones given to cattle to increase the growth of lean meat and to reduce feeding costs can promote cancer.

bST, developed to increase milk production in cows, is not currently approved for use in this country, but It is currently under FDA review. Dr. Hotchkiss believes that this type of hormone "is of no concern" to consumers primarily because it is a protein and like all proteins it is broken down

Commonly Used Food Additives Approved by FDA

	Examples	Found In	Comments
Colors	FD&C certified colors, annatto, carotene chlorophyll, cochineal	Baked goods, soft drinks, cheeses, ice cream, sherbet, caramel cake mixes, candy	Of the 33 colors approved for use in foods, only 7 are synthetically produced (FD&C colors) yet they account for most food coloring used today.
Flavor & flavor enhancers	Salt, caffeine, flavorings, vanilla, herbs, spices, ammoniated glycyrrhizin, MSG, maltol, hydrolyzed vegetable protein	Soda and fruit drinks, pie filling, gelatin, candy, ice cream, preserves, cookies, baked goods, soup, seafood, poultry, cheese, sauces, frankfurters	Flavors are the largest single category of food additives. Approximately 1,700 natural and synthetically derived flavoring compounds are permitted for use in foods.
Sweeteners	Sugar, fructose, corn syrup, sorbitol, saccharin, aspartame, acesulfame-K	Soft drinks, candies, gum, baked goods, frozen desserts	Sweeteners are the most controversial of flavoring substances. Although FDA tried to ban saccharin because animals fed large doses developed bladder tumors, consumer demand forced FDA to permit its use. Aspartame (*NutraSweet*) has reportedly caused headaches and dizziness. Concerns about acesulfame-K have also been raised.

in the human digestive tract to its component amino acids.

Government Regulation of Food Additives. Although several Federal agencies share responsibility for regulating food additives, the FDA takes the leading role. The Delaney Clause—part of legislation passed in 1958—prohibits the use of any substance, which in any amount, causes cancer in animals or humans. But, food safety experts and food manufacturers have sharply criticized the Delaney Clause in recent years as being too rigid and impractical.

Opponents argue that the law has not kept pace with the advances in analytical chemistry, which have all allowed scientists to detect ex-

traordinarily minute quantities of food components down to one part per billion (ppb). In monetary terms, 1 ppb would be the equivalent of 1 cent in $10 million dollars.

In addition, Delaney detractors point out that the law does not take into account the risk posed by *not* using some additives considered harmful (e.g. nitrites in cured meats which prevent the growth of bacterium that cause botulism, a deadly food poison).

Additive Risks. Risk taking is inescapable. Consumers face risks daily, from crossing the street to flying in a plane. While it is undeniable that certain food additives are potential threats to health, food safety experts emphasize that Americans should put the risk into proper perspective. For example, it is estimated that diet and tobacco together account for about 67% of cancer deaths, while all chemicals in food including pesticide residues pose less than a 1% risk.

Even Michael Jacobson, Ph.D. Executive Director of the Center for Science in the Public Interest, and an outspoken critic of food additives agrees that "there are much bigger risks than food additives, like driving without seat belts, eating fatty foods and drinking alcoholic beverages." While Jacobson agrees with food safety experts who say that the risks additives pose to individual consumers is small, he disagrees with them regarding the risk additives pose to society. He argues that even a minuscule risk when multiplied by millions of people results in a significant and intolerable risk, especially when an additive does not perform an essential function.

The Bottom Line. While Americans enjoy the safest food supply in the world, many feel it could be made even safer. What to do now? If exposure to food additives is a concern, first and foremost, eat a variety of foods to limit exposure to any single additive, focusing on fresh, minimally processed foods. Limit intake of artificial colors by reading labels. The specific color may not be listed, but the ingredient list should say "artificially colored." Reading labels is especially important for the small segment of the population sensitive to specific additives such as yellow #5.

—*Ira Milner, R.D.*

Source: *Environmental Nutrition,* Vol. 12, No. 11, November 1989.

If fast foods are a regular part of your life-style, steps can be taken to make up for their shortcomings. To cut back on fat and refined sugar, choose low-fat milk or fruit juice rather than soft drinks and shakes. Processed cheese, pickles, and salted french fries contain much sodium, so choose selectively. The sauce on burgers is also high in fat. Ask that sauce and pickles be left off, and that fries not be salted. Skip the deep-fried desserts and soft ice cream. Pizza can be a good choice. It is lower in fat than many other fast foods, although it is high in sodium (and skip the pepperoni and sausage in favor of vegetable toppings). Salad bars and baked potatoes are nutritious additions to fast-food establishments. Salad bar toppings and the stuffings for potatoes can be high in fat or sodium, so choose with discretion.

Balance a day that includes a fast-food meal, by including in other meals, fresh fruits and vegetables, whole grains, and whole wheat bread, and limit foods high in sodium and fat. An occasional fast-food meal can be part of a nutritious diet. The key, as always, is moderation and keeping an appropriate balance.

Do We Need To Take Nutritional Supplements?
The increased popularity of nutritional supplements is part of the move towards greater self-responsibility for health and the recognition that nutrition is an important facet of well-being. Unfor-

tunately, much misinformation and many misplaced expectations have surrounded the rise of the nutrition in a pill approach to health. Americans are now spending $3 billion a year on vitamins, a sixfold increase during the past 15 years. Their sellers work hard to convince us we need supplements to improve our health, sex life, athletic abilities, stress level, and longevity. Estimates of how many adults use supplements range from 36 percent to 55 percent of the population, and the average money spent per user is estimated at $32 annually (6, 10).

Supplements are clearly useful for meeting nutritional needs for those with special physical conditions. These include anemia, pregnancy, intolerance to milk, and use of certain medications such as oral contraceptives. In addition, if one has been consuming less than 1500 calories, a diet high in processed foods, or has a poorly balanced diet, many nutritionists and dietitians recommend individuals take a balanced vitamin/mineral supplement that provides nutrients at RDA levels.

Are there other justifications for taking supplements? The debate goes back and forth. Some people feel that with the lengthy storage and transportation of food resulting in nutrient losses, and consumption of the many processed and refined foods, we can no longer be assured that we will obtain the nutrients we need from food. We should, they believe, use supplements as "insurance." Others argue that through wise food choices and minimizing nutrient losses during storage and preparation we can nourish ourselves quite well without them. Still others say high-potency nutrient supplements have only recently become available; since the body has evolved genetically utilizing the nutrients obtained from food, not isolated chemicals, we should be cautious, they say, in taking doses greater than the amounts present naturally in the diet.

Is there a problem in taking supplements if they're not really needed? When a nutrient is taken in amounts much larger than those present naturally in the diet, normal nutrient pathways in the body become saturated. The nutrient spills over into other pathways and may act like a drug. Taken in these pharmacological amounts, risk of side effects is present, as with any drug. For example, vitamin A toxicity can occur when 10 times the RDA is taken daily over time and results in dry skin, headache, nausea, vomiting, joint pain, hair loss, anorexia, and enlarged liver and spleen. Nutrient balances can also be affected, since an excess of one nutrient can interfere with normal metabolism of another. Large amounts of zinc, for example, interfere with copper absorption in the intestine, potentially creating a copper deficiency. Also

(continued on p. 152)

Seeking a Nutrition Counselor? How To Tell the Pros from the Quacks

Today, among Californians particularly, it's the "in" thing to have a "personal nutritionist." With the elevation of health and fitness to status symbols, it's become a matter of self-esteem to have a nutrition counselor to call one's own. Unhappily, few people seem to realize how common it is to hear disreputable, unreliable, unethical and in some cases even dangerous advice from self-proclaimed "nutritionists."

Charlatans can be found anywhere: in health clubs, in chiropractors' offices, dentists' offices, even physicians' offices. The doctor himself may be giving unreliable nutrition advice. Some well-known syndicated newspaper columnists and radio show hosts who have questionable credentials have jumped on the bandwagon too.

So, how can the average person choose an individual who is a reliable source of nutrition advice? Here's what to look for and what to avoid when seeking a nutrition counselor:

Beware of Meaningless Titles and Credentials. Anyone can hang out a shingle and call herself or himself a nutritionist, nutrition counselor or nutrition advisor, regardless of credentials.

The title R.D., which stands for registered dietitian, can only be used by people who have met professional criteria, including a four-year degree from an accredited college or university, plus either a six to 12 month internship in a hospital or clinic, or a master's degree and six months of work experience as a dietitian.

Furthermore, to obtain the right to use (and keep) the R.D. title, the individual must pass a national exam and accumulate at least 75 hours of continuing nutrition education every five years.

While the R.D. credential can't absolutely insure the best advice, it is the easiest and most reliable way to screen out unqualified or disreputable individuals.

A responsible, qualified nutritionist SHOULD:

- Individualize a diet plan for each person's unique needs, taking into consideration current eating habits, lifestyle and medical history.
- Focus *first* on modifying eating habits to maximize nutrition, *then* turn to vitamin and mineral supplements if needs cannot be met by diet alone.
- Encourage a diet that's low in fat, high in complex carbohydrates and fiber, and moderate in sodium, sugar and alcohol.
- Be realistic by working into the diet plan an individual's favorite foods, occasional dining out and snacks.
- Encourage exercise and suggest behavior modification techniques when counseling clients on weight-loss diets.
- Consult with the client's personal physician if under medical care.
- Encourage a wide variety of foods.

A responsible, qualified nutritionist should NOT:

- Promise or attempt to cure chronic diseases.
- Attribute common and vague symptoms to a disorder such as hypoglycemia, food allergies or malabsorption, and then claim that diet is the answer.
- Evaluate vitamin/mineral or general nutritional status by hair analysis, iridology (tear drop tests) or other unproven methods.
- Sell nutrient supplements after recommending that clients take them.
- Promise fast, effortless and easy weight loss.
- Hand out pre-printed diets without individual counseling.
- Recommend a diet with less than 1,000 calories a day, except in extreme cases and then only under a physician's supervision and continual monitoring.

Few states have legal standards governing the word "nutritionist," though 16 states have recently licensed dietitians (L.D.). Like R.D.'s, licensed dietitians are required to meet stringent educational and professional standards.

Look Out for Bogus Degrees. There are persons other than R.D.'s and L.D.'s who are qualified to give nutrition counseling, but it may be a bit trickier to sort out the good from the bad. An M.S. or Ph.D. after a name may look impressive but may be irrelevant if the degree happens to be in English literature, for example. Even the initials M.D. after someone's name don't guarantee good information. Some of the best-selling diet books with the most inaccurate information have been written by M.D.'s.

A person offering to act as a nutrition counselor but who is not an R.D. should at least have a degree in nutrition or dietetics from an accredited college or university. Check with the state board of education to be sure that the program is accredited.

A non-R.D. whose undergraduate degree is limited, for example, to a related field such as biology, should have a graduate degree in nutrition. As an additional check, see if the person is a member of the following professional associations:

- American College of Nutrition
- American Dietetic Association
- American Institute of Nutrition
- American Society of Clinical Nutrition
- Society for Nutrition Education

There are several institutions claiming to offer "degrees" in nutrition and nutrition counseling, which, in fact, are worth little more than the paper they're printed on! Three such institutions are: American College of Health Science in Texas; American Nutrimedical University in Indiana; and Donsbach University in California.

Recognize Proper Professional Counseling. Good health depends on many factors—nutrition is only one. Don't expect changes in diet alone to miraculously cure or prevent any illness. Be suspicious of anyone who suggests that they will.

—*Susan Male Smith, M.S., R.D.*

Source: *Environmental Nutrition,* Vol. 10, No. 11, November 1987.

---

of concern is contamination of supplements. As an example, 13 people in 15 states during the course of 1984 developed selenium toxicity after taking selenium supplements that contained more than 180 times the amount specified on the label and considered safe (11). Samples of spirulina algae powder have contained mercury concentrations above allowable limits (7).

Although the debate will continue, nutritionists are generally in agreement that no harm will come from using a balanced vitamin-mineral supplement supplying nutrients at RDA levels (8). In fact, a survey found that 60 percent of Washington state dietitians, professionals well-versed in nutritional needs and dietary intakes, used supplements (9). If you are considering a nutrient supplement for a specific need, consult a qualified nutritionist, dietitian, or physician specializing in nutrition. And regardless of one's stance on the issue, everyone agrees that use of supplements in no way decreases the need for a nutritious diet.

(continued on p. 155)

Finding a diet, nutrition or cook book is easy; most bookstores have large sections devoted to eating (or not eating, as the case may be). What isn't so easy is finding one that is accurate, practical and reliable.

Books devoted to the topic of eating appear regularly on best seller lists. But replacing the old standby diet books now are new nutrition books concerned with maintaining good health by eating right. And new specialized books also zero in on how nutrition affects specific diseases. Evidently, it's no longer possible to write a bestseller merely about losing 10, 20 or even 30 pounds. The new wave of books embraces good nutrition as a lifestyle, acknowledging that nutrition is a complex science of interrelationships. But the sophistication of the new books create a new problem: it's more difficult now—even for professionals—to distinguish the good books from the bad. Readers must be more knowledgeable than ever before when choosing.

Choosing a Reliable Nutrition Book: Tips to Take to the Bookstore

Many people assume they are protected from inaccurate or misleading information; that if it's in print, the information must be correct. In fact, authors are protected by the first amendment and can say whatever they wish, as long as it is not libellous.

With a few guidelines, however, the average reader can learn how to separate the wheat from the chaff and come away with a few golden grains of nutrition knowledge. Below are *Environmental Nutrition's* tips on how to guard against being duped and how to choose worthwhile nutrition reading.

Meanwhile, it's encouraging to know that there *are* good nutrition books being published. But they are far outnumbered by bad ones on the best seller list. All the more reason then, to use these guidelines. Look beyond the sensational hype to find good, basic, reliable nutrition advice. It's worth the extra time.

—*Susan Male Smith, M.A., R.D.*

YES, DO LOOK FOR A BOOK THAT:

- *Follows the United States Dietary Guidelines: high in complex carbohydrates, low in fat and moderate in protein.* This translates to lots of whole grains, fruits and vegetables, no more than six ounces of meat a day, and only low-fat or fat-free dairy products. High fiber foods should be embraced gradually, but excessive salt, sugar and alcohol should be discouraged.
- *Encourages a variety of foods.* Few items should be taboo. Rather, smaller portions of a few high-calorie foods should be suggested as a way to cut calories.
- *Promotes life-long changes* in eating, not just a two-or three-week "diet."

- *Encourages a gradual approach* to new eating habits. Changes made too fast are doomed to failure. Better to change one thing at a time and make it last.
- *Give practical suggestions* for incorporating dietary changes into everyday life, including meal planning, shopping, preparation, eating out and special occasions.
- *Encourages regular exercise* to keep fit and provides specifics on how to start slowly and keep motivated.
- *Uses language that is easy to read and understand.* A good book doesn't get bogged down in technical detail, and it often provides a helpful glossary of complicated terms.
- *Provides scientific references* when research is cited.
- *Advises the reader to see a physician* before making significant changes in his or her diet.

NO, DON'T BUY OR READ A BOOK THAT:

- *Promises to cure a disease.* Many conditions may be improved or controlled by diet; some might even be prevented or delayed. But none—except outright nutrient deficiencies—can be cured.
- *Promises fast results.* A weight loss of more than two or three pounds a week is not fat, but water, or worse, lean muscle tissue. The weight is easily gained back as soon as the diet is liberalized or forsaken. Some research even suggests that lost lean weight may be gained back as fat!
- *Emphasizes one or two food groups,* to the exclusion of others. A good diet encourages eating a variety of foods.
- *Promotes the idea that certain combinations of foods are harmful.* Healthy people can digest proteins, carbohydrates and fats at the same time with no problem. In fact, most foods are a natural combination of these components.
- *Encourages megadoses of vitamins and minerals.* With a varied diet of 1400 calories or more, supplements shouldn't be necessary. At any rate, there are few instances in which anyone needs to take more than 100 percent of the RDA. Before doing so, they should see a physician. Unbalanced nutrient supplementation can interfere with the absorption and utilization of other nutrients and medications.
- *Denigrates traditional medicine* and the need for scientific research, while promoting the "conspiracy theory," i.e., that the information in the book is being withheld from the public by the medical community.
- *Advises readers to ignore side effects* resulting from following the book's advice. Side effects should never be ignored.
- *Relies on personal testimonials,* instead of scientific evidence.

Source: *Environmental Nutrition,* Vol. 11, No. 6, June 1988.

How to Decide What to Believe

Determining whether nutritional information is truthful or misleading is not an easy task. Popular nutrition books and magazine articles can be full of sincere but misguided, incomplete, or out-of-context information.

We live in an age in which cancer, heart disease, and other chronic diseases have affected our own circle of family and friends. The era of wonder drugs has left us with the hope that potent drugs will continue to solve whatever ails us or new substances will be discovered to push our bodies to their ultimate potential. The advertisers and authors of best-selling health and diet books know we want to believe the information they give us and they make it hard for us not to. Without closing our minds to new approaches and new information, it is equally important, in the age of the fast megabuck, to interpret what we read critically and with a healthy dose of skepticism, to be aware of the financial motivations involved, and to acknowledge the vulnerable and easily exploited nature of the human spirit of hope (see the boxes "Seeking a Nutrition Counselor? How to Tell the Pros from the Quacks" and "Choosing a Reliable Nutrition Book: Tips to Take to the Bookstore").

Did You Know That . . .

What may seem like a light and nonfattening treat, a croissant contains 50 percent more calories and 12 times as much fat as an English muffin of the same weight.

GUIDING PRINCIPLES
FOR DIETARY CHANGE

We have looked at many of the pros and cons of the American diet. We have seen that Americans tend to consume too few foods high in complex carbohydrate, fiber, vitamins, and minerals. On average, Americans also consume too many refined and processed foods, and foods high in fat, sodium, and sugar.

A few important concepts deserve reemphasis to guide us through the maze of nutritional recommendations we have explored: variety, moderation, unprocessed foods, and gradual, enjoyable change.

Variety

Mangos, pistachios, jicama root, bean sprouts, onion bagels, goat cheese, Cuban black beans, squid, kiwi fruit, hot chili salsa—a world of exotic flavors is all around us. Traditional American foods are just as full of variety and taste—pumpkin pie, baked apples, sweet potatoes, chicken and dumplings, rice pudding, zucchini fritters, fried green tomatoes, Boston baked beans, buttermilk pancakes.

In spite of the thousands of items lining grocery store shelves, Americans tend to consume too little a variety of foods. Eating many different foods provides us with the 50 or so nutrients we need and minimizes chances of overconsuming one nutrient or contaminant to unhealthy levels. And with so many delicious foods available, why forgo the pleasures they offer? The first guideline for a nutritious diet, then, is to include many different types of foods in our diet.

Moderation

The old saying encouraging moderation in all things is particularly applicable to nutrition. There is no food we should absolutely never have. The idea is rather to eat less frequently or in smaller portions those foods that are less nutritious. For example, a piece of chocolate cake every day may provide too much fat and sugar if someone's diet is already a little high in these ingredients. A piece now and then, however, can fit easily into a healthy diet.

Portion size is also a part of moderation. A 4-ounce steak provides plenty of protein and important minerals. A 10-ounce steak probably provides too much saturated fat in a single meal. Good nutrition is not an all or nothing affair, but a matter of emphasizing some foods more than others, some foods less.

Whole and Unprocessed Foods

By eating foods in their original state we incorporate many important nutritional recommendations at once. Most unprocessed foods are low in sodium, sugar, and fat. They contain fiber and nutrients missing in refined versions. When unprocessed foods are the foundation of the diet, an occasional excursion into less nutritious food choices is not likely to harm health. An added plus of whole foods is lower cost. A serving of oatmeal costs pennies, while a serving of highly refined, presweetened and ready-to-eat cereal costs 10 times as much.

Gradual and Enjoyable Change

A healthy diet is important, but a relaxed attitude about food is equally important. For mental and physical well-being we need foods that are nutritious and that we enjoy. When we focus on the "don'ts" of nutrition, eating becomes a task rather than a joy. Instead, focus on small changes that are simple and easy. If we add a glass of low-fat milk to lunch, we might find we have consumed one less soft drink during the day without even thinking about it. If we add an extra serving of bread to dinner, we might find we don't have room for a second serving of meat. Thus, less healthy old patterns and preferences pass away quietly and are replaced by new ones.

In addition to making changes that are enjoyed, moving slowly is important. We cannot overhaul ourselves overnight. We may want to make major changes in our diet, but if they are attempted too abruptly we're likely to feel deprived, give in, and end up where we started. Slow, gradual, pleasant changes are the ones likely to stay. Once a change has become second nature, we are ready to work on the next one.

The challenge in developing a healthy diet is to achieve balance, not to follow hard and fast rules. Like a row of dominos gently tapped at one end, making small changes in one area of the diet causes other areas to shift into place almost effortlessly at the same time.

PLAN OF ACTION

New, health-promoting food choices can be as simple as switching from whole milk to low-fat milk or buying whole wheat bread half of the time. But you may be wondering where to start!

1. Begin by observing your current patterns. Keep a record of what and when you eat for a few days. Then look at it carefully. When do you eat and how often? What kinds of foods do you eat? How often do you drink coffee, eat sweets and fats, or eat whole grain foods? Do you see consistent patterns that merit changing? How can you improve your diet?

2. Choose one aspect of your diet to work on—something small and specific. Examples are cutting back on the meat portion at dinner, eating fresh fruit in place of a soft drink in the afternoon, consuming breakfast if you weren't before, etc. If your family has a history of high blood cholesterol, you may want to cut back on saturated fat consumption. If a fast-paced, heavy-on-the-coffee life-style is making you stressed and nervous, you might start with reducing caffeine consumption.

3. Plan ahead. Determine specific times of the day to implement your change and have the appropriate foods available. For example, carry fruit with you during the day to replace sweet or salty snacks. A goal to eat more salads is of no avail if you

forget to keep lettuce on hand. Do you need the cooperation of family members or roommates if meals are shared? Discuss your plans to gain their support. Assess your environment. Know where the foods you want are available during the day.

4. Seek additional help and resources if necessary. School health centers often have nutrition counselors. Visit a bookstore for nutrition books and cookbooks. Nutritionists and dietitians in private practice can help you plan general dietary improvements, diets for optimal sports performance, or diets for special needs. Nutrition instructors at local colleges and extension home economists are sources of information about foods, cooking, and nutrition. Local community education programs may offer low-fat cooking classes. Most colleges offer introductory courses in nutrition.

Keep in mind the key to successful change is to choose an area you *want* to change and are motivated to do so. There is no need to force too big or too quick a change. In time, your new, healthier habits will become your preferred ones. Be patient—allow time for this process of a long-term, enjoyable change to take place. Ⓦ

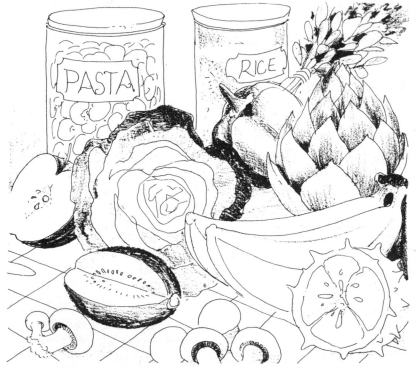

Glossary

A

Adaptive thermogenesis: Exercise and restrictive eating which results in the total number of calories burned in a day.

Aerobic exercise: Exercise in which the body is able to meet the muscles' increased demand for oxygen continuously during increased activity. Aerobic means "requiring air to live."

Amino acids: Nitrogen-containing compounds that are the building blocks of proteins. Twenty-two amino acids occur in proteins.

Atherosclerosis: A form of hardening of the arteries in which lipids and calcium plaques gradually accumulate on artery walls, causing the blood vessels to lose elasticity and the arterial openings to narrow.

B

Basal metabolic rate: The energy required to keep the body functioning at rest (to maintain breathing, heartbeat, body temperature, and other bodily functions).

Beta-carotene: A water-soluble compound found in fruits and vegetables that is transformed into vitamin A by the body.

Bile acids: Liquids secreted by the liver to carry away waste products formed in the liver. It helps break down fats in the small intestine during digestion.

Blood cholesterol: Cholesterol found in the blood and made by the liver from a wide variety of foods, especially saturated fats.

C

Caffeinism: A response to an overdose of caffeine that resembles an anxiety attack with dizziness, agitation, sleep difficulties, restlessness, and headache.

Calorie: Technically, a unit used to measure energy equivalent to the amount of heat that raises the temperature of 1 gram of water 1 degree centigrade. Calories in food represent the energy value of the food, and are measured in kilocalories (a thousand calories), although in common usage we refer to these kilocalories simply as calories.

Carcinogen: Any agent capable of causing cancer. The three broad categories are chemical, which includes tobacco smoke, physical, which includes X-rays, and biological, which includes certain viruses.

Cholesterol: A fatlike substance found in animal foods and also manufactured by the body. It is essential to nerve and brain cell function, the synthesis of sex hormones, and is a component of bile acids used to aid fat digestion. Cholesterol is also a part of atherosclerotic plaques that accumulate on artery walls.

Complementary proteins: A term used to signify protein foods that together provide a complete set of essential amino acids, such as beans and a corn tortilla.

Complex carbohydrate: A polysaccharide, or compound consisting of many sugar molecules linked together. Complex carbohydrates in the diet include starches and the fiber, cellulose.

Coronary artery disease (CAD): Disease of the arteries that supply blood to the heart muscle, causing damage to, or malfunction of, the heart.

Couscous: A North African dish consisting of steamed semolina served with meat and vegetables.

D

Delaney Clause: A clause in the Food, Drug, and Cosmetic Act which states that no substance known to cause cancer in animals or humans at any dose shall be added to foods.

Diabetes: A disorder in which the pancreas produces insufficient or no insulin, the hormone responsible for the absorption of glucose into the cells for energy.

Dietary cholesterol: Cholesterol added to the body's natural cholesterol through the food one eats.

Diuretic: A compound that stimulates increased excretion of water via the kidneys.

E

Enriched: The addition of nutrients to foods that have lost nutrients during the process of refining. Enriched flour contains additions of niacin, riboflavin, thiamin, and iron in amounts similar to those originally present in the whole grain.

Enzyme: A protein compound that facilitates biochemical reactions.

Epidemiology: The study of disease as it affects groups of people, as opposed to individuals.

Essential amino acids: The 9 amino acids the body cannot form from other nitrogen-containing compounds and which must be obtained through the diet. They are phenylalanine, valine, threonine, tryptophan, isoleucine, methionine, histidine, leucine, and lysine.

F

Fat-soluble vitamins: Vitamins that are found in the fatty portions of foods and that can be stored in the body. Vitamins A, E, and D are fat-soluble.

Fatty acid: Chemical compounds containing carbon, hydrogen, and oxygen. They form part of the triglycerides in food and in the body and can be saturated, polyunsaturated, or monounsaturated.

FD&C Red # 3: Food additive used primarily to color maraschino and cocktail cherries and pistachio nuts; claiming it to be an animal carcinogen, the Public Citizen Litigation Group is fighting to have it banned.

Food additive: Natural and chemical substances added to foods to enhance flavor and color and act as a preservative.

Fortified: The addition of nutrients to foods in amounts greater than those naturally present in the food. Breakfast cereals and milk are foods that are most often fortified.

Fructose: A monosaccharide or simple sugar, often referred to as fruit sugar. It is also found in honey and is part of the disaccharide sucrose, or table sugar.

G

Galactose: A monosaccharide or simple sugar; part of the disaccharide lactose found in milk.

Glucose: A monosaccharide or simple sugar found in foods by itself and also as part of complex carbohydrates and the disaccharides sucrose, maltose, and lactose; also known as blood sugar.

Glycogen: A form of complex carbohydrate stored in the body. It is found primarily in liver and muscle tissue.

H

HDL (High-density lipoproteins): Lipoproteins that return cholesterol to the liver for processing and excretion.

Heme iron: The deep red iron-containing chemical constituent of hemoglobin; it is found primarily in meat.

Hydrogenation: A process of adding hydrogen to unsaturated fatty acids to make them more saturated and solid.

Hyperactivity: A behavior pattern of certain children who are constantly overactive and have difficulty concentrating on one activity.

Hypertension: Abnormally high blood pressure at rest.

Hypoglycemia: An abnormally low level of glucose in the blood usually caused by the concurrent condition of diabetes.

I

Incomplete protein: The protein, considered incomplete because it doesn't contain all 9 essential amino acids, that is found in legumes, grains, and vegetables.

Indole: A compound of decomposing proteins containing tryptophan.

Insulin: A hormone produced by the pancreas in varying amounts depending on the level of blood sugar; it promotes the absorption of glucose into the liver and into muscle cells.

Insoluble fiber: Fiber incapable of being dissolved in a liquid.

K

Kasha: A mush made usually from buckwheat groats.

L

Lactation: The secretion of milk.

Lacto-ovo-vegetarians: A vegetarian diet that allows milk, eggs, and milk products such as cheese, but excludes all types of fish, poultry, and red meat.

LDL (Low-density lipoproteins): Lipoproteins that contain large amounts of cholesterol which they carry through the blood stream and deposit in cells.

Legumes: Dried beans and peas such as pinto, kidney, black, and navy beans. Legumes are rich in B vitamins, protein, and complex carbohydrates.

Lipoproteins: A compound of protein and lipids manufactured by the liver which moves cholesterol throughout the body.

Lymphatic system: A network of vessels and ducts that transport and hold fluid in the interstitial space, the area between blood vessels and cells.

M

Macronutrients: A large quantity (over a gram) of nutrients essential to growth and health.

Mammary: A gland in the female breast that can produce milk.

Metabolic rate: The energy required to keep the body functioning at rest (to maintain breathing, heartbeat, body temperature, and other bodily functions). The metabolic rate increases in response to exertion, stress, fear, and illness. Also known as basal metabolic rate.

Micronutrients: Organic compounds, such as vitamins, essential in minute amounts (less than a gram) to growth and health.

Monounsaturated fat: A type of triglyceride, rich in monounsaturated fatty acids such as oleic acid, that contains only one point of unsaturation in its chemical structure. Olive, peanut, and canola oils are rich in monounsaturated fats.

N

Neurotransmitters: Chemical messengers in the brain that are released from the ends of nerve cells.

Nirvana: A place or state of mind in which one is oblivious to care, pain, or external reality.

Nonheme iron: The iron found primarily in legumes, grains, and vegetables; it is less easily absorbed by the body than heme iron.

Nutrients: Compounds used by the body for growth, maintenance, and repair. Nutrients are essential to life and most cannot be manufactured by the body and must be taken in through food.

O

Omega-3 fatty acids: Polyunsaturated fats found in fish oils and important in synthesis of hormonelike prostaglandins.

Osteoporosis: A condition of weak, porous bones resulting from loss of bone density over time.

P

Pellagra: A nutritional disorder caused by a deficiency of niacin (vitamin B complex) resulting in dermatitis, diarrhea, and dementia.

Pernicious anemia: A type of anemia caused by failure to absorb vitamin B_{12}, which is essential for normal red blood cell production in the bone marrow.

Polyunsaturated fat: A type of triglyceride rich in polyunsaturated fatty acids such as linoleic and linolenic acid that contains several points of unsaturation in its chemical structure. Safflower, soy, corn, sesame, cottonseed, and sunflower oils are rich in polyunsaturated fatty acids.

Processed food: A food that has been treated by canning, freezing, fortification, enrichment, refining, or a change in texture.

Prostaglandins: hormonelike compounds synthesized in the body from fatty acids with roles in numerous body processes.

R

Recommended Dietary Allowances (RDAs): The amount of vitamins, minerals, protein, and energy that is necessary for humans to ingest daily to maintain health and energy.

Retinol: The chief and typical vitamin A.

Riboflavin: Also referred to as vitamin B_2, it is one of the B complex vitamins important in the metabolism of energy nutrients.

S

Saturated fat: A type of triglyceride rich in saturated fatty acids such as stearic acid that contain no points of unsaturation in their chemical structure. Animal foods, palm oil, and coconut oil are rich in saturated fats.

Scurvy: A disease caused by inadequate intake of vitamin C and characterized by weakness of the blood vessels causing bleeding anywhere in the body.

Semi-vegetarian: A vegetarian diet that includes milk, eggs, milk products such as cheese and cream, and allows occasional fish and poultry but no red meat.

Serotonin: A neurotransmitter in the brain formed from the amino acid tryptophan that may have a role in modulating sleep and pain.

Serum cholesterol: Cholesterol found in the clear fluid that separates from blood when it clots.

Soluble fiber: Fiber capable of being dissolved in fluid.

Sucrose: A dissaccharide, or sugar composed of two component sugar molecules, glucose and fructose, found in table sugar, beet sugar, and cane sugar.

T

Thermic effect of feeding: The number of calories needed to digest food and store nutrients.

Threshold point: The point at which a physiological or psychological effect, such as pain, begins to be produced.

Trace minerals: Minerals in the body in very small quantities, each amounting to less than a total of 5 grams.

Transfatty acids: "Mirror image" molecules produced during the hydrogenation of unsaturated fatty acids.

Triglyceride: A fat compound found in foods and made in the body, consisting of a carbon "backbone" to which are attached three fatty acids.

U

Unsaturated fats: The general category of fats that has one or several points on the carbon atom unoccupied by hydrogen. If one point is unoccupied, it is considered monounsaturated; if several points are unoccupied, it is considered polyunsaturated. Vegetable fats are unsaturated in varying degrees.

V

Vegans: Strict vegetarians who abstain from eating animal foods as well as dairy products and eggs.

Vitamins: Organic (carbon-containing) compounds essential to life and needed in very small quantities. They are nutrients not made by the body and so must be obtained from food.

W

Water-soluble vitamins: Vitamins that are found in the watery compartments of foods and the body; excreted in the urine if body concentrations become too high. The B-complex vitamins and vitamin C are water-soluble.

Y

Yellow # 5: Food additive that may cause allergic reactions in some people; required by law to be named on product labels.

Notes

CHAPTER 1

1. Committee on Diet and Health, Food and Nutrition Board, Commission on Life Sciences, National Research Council, "Dietary Intake and Nutritional Status: Trends and Assessment," *Diet and Health: Implications For Reducing Chronic Disease Risk* (Washington, DC: National Academy Press, 1989), 41–84.
2. "The Healthy Eater's Guide To Sugar," *University of California, Berkeley Wellness Letter* 6, no. 3 (1989): 4–5.
3. K. Morgan, V. Stults, and G. Stampley, "Soft Drink Consumption Patterns of the U.S. Population," *Journal of the American Dietetic Association* 3 (1985): 352–354.
4. U.S. Senate Select Committee on Nutrition and Human Needs, *Dietary Goals For the United States* (Washington, DC: Government Printing Office, 1977).
5. Committee on Diet and Health, pp. 55–59.
6. Letitia Brewster and Michael Jacobsen, "Foods in our Diet," in *The Changing American Diet* (Washington, DC: Center for Science in the Public Interest, 1979), 3–4.
7. "The Soft Drink Explosion," *Nutrition Action* 8, no. 7 (1981): 8.
8. Brewster and Jacobsen, p. 60.
9. Jane Brody, *Jane Brody's Nutrition Book* (New York: Bantam Books, 1987), 14.
10. A. C. Nielson, *Who's Dieting and Why?* (Chicago, IL: A. C. Nielson Co., 1979).
11. Brody, p. 16.

CHAPTER 2

1. U.S Department of Agriculture, *Nationwide Food Consumption Survey. Nutrient Intakes: Individuals in 48 States, Year 1977–1978*, Report No. I–2 (Hyattsville, MD: Consumer Nutrition Division, Human Nutrition Information Services, 1984).
2. Department of Health, Education, and Welfare, *Ten-State Nutrition Survey 1968–1970*, vols. I–VI, DHEW Publication No. HSM-72-8130, 72-8132, 72-8133, 72-8134 (Atlanta, GA: Center for Disease Control, Health Services and Mental Health Administration).

3. U.S. Department of Health and Human Services/Department of Agriculture, *Nutrition Monitoring in the United States—A Progress Report from the Joint Nutrition Monitoring Evaluation Committee*, DHHS Publication No. (PHS) 86-1255, (Hyattsville, MD: National Center for Health Statistics, 1987).

4. Committee on Dietary Allowances, Food and Nutrition Board, National Research Council, *Recommended Dietary Allowances*, 10th ed. (Washington, DC: National Academy of Sciences Press, 1989).

5. J. King et al., "Evaluation and Modification of the Basic Four Food Guide," *Journal of Nutrition Education* 10 (1978): 27–29.

6. P. Hausman, "Updating the Basic Four," *Nutrition Action* 6, no. 1 (1979): 8–9.

7. Alice Chenault, *Nutrition and Health* (New York: Holt, Rinehart & Winston, 1984), 46–53.

8. U.S. Department of Agriculture and U.S. Department of Health, Education, and Welfare, *Nutrition and Your Health: Dietary Guidelines For Americans* (Washington, DC: Government Printing Office, 1980).

9. Committee on Diet and Health, pp. 3–22.

10. National Cancer Institute, U.S. Department of Health and Human Services, *Diet, Nutrition, and Cancer Prevention: A Guide To Food Choices*, NIH Publication No. 85-2711 (Washington, DC: Government Printing Office, 1985).

CHAPTER 3

1. George Briggs and Doris Calloway, *Nutrition and Physical Fitness* 11th ed. (New York: Holt, Rinehart & Winston, 1984), 124.

2. Committee on Dietary Allowances, pp. 32–36.

3. Committee on Diet and Health, pp. 16, 114–115.

4. "Exercise Burns Calories in More Ways Than One," *Tufts University Diet and Nutrition Letter* 7, no. 10 (1989): 2.

5. C. Madden, "What Keeps Obese Persons Obese?" *Canadian Association of Health, Physical Education, and Recreation Journal* (July-August, 1983): 5–7.

6. P. Sorlie, T. Gordon, and W. Kannel, "Body Build and Mortality: The Framingham Study," *Journal of the American Medical Association* 248, no. 18 (1980): 1828.

7. "Feeling Fat in a Thin Society," *Glamour*, 1984, 198–201, 251–252.

8. Briggs and Calloway, p. 36.

9. Committee on Diet and Health, pp. 15–16.
10. "Chromium Deficiency May Increase Risk of Diabetes," *Environmental Nutrition* 11, no. 3 (1988): 1–3.
11. R. A. Anderson, "Chromium Metabolism and Its Role in Disease Processes in Man," *Clinical Physical Biochemistry* 4 (1986): 31–41.
12. "The Healthy Eater's Guide To Sugar," *University of California Wellness Letter* 6, no. 3 (1989): 4–5.
13. Committee on Diet and Health, p. 58.
14. U.S. Department of Agriculture, *Dietary Guidelines for Americans.*
15. Committee on Diet and Health, pp. 291–309.
16. E. Lanza et al., "A Critical Review of Food Fiber Analysis and Data," *Journal of the American Dietetic Association* 86 (1986): 732–743.
17. U.S. Senate Select Committee on Nutrition and Human Needs, *Dietary Goals For the United States* (Washington, DC: Government Printing Office, 1977).
18. U.S. Senate Select Committee on Nutrition and Human Needs.
19. Committee on Diet and Health, pp. 682–683.

CHAPTER 4

1. Chenault, p. 100.
2. Eleanor Hamilton and Eva May Whitney, *Nutrition Concepts and Controversies* (St. Paul, MN: West Publishing, 1982), 169.
3. "Protein Overload," *University of California, Berkeley Wellness Letter* 5, no. 12 (1989): 6.
4. Committee on Diet and Health, pp. 15–16.
5. Chenault, p. 117.
6. M. Zaidins, "Is Public Interest in Fish Fading? Reasons Why It Shouldn't," *Environmental Nutrition* 12, no. 4 (1989): 1–3.
7. Frances Moore Lappe, *Diet for a Small Planet,* (New York: Ballentine Books, 1982), 66–88.
8. "Lessons We Can Learn from Vegetarians," *Tufts University Diet and Nutrition Letter* 6, no. 5 (1988): 3–6.
9. Sonja Conner and William E. Conner, *The New American Diet* (New York: Simon & Schuster, 1986), 96.
10. "Heart Facts," American Heart Association, 1985.
11. National Cholesterol Education Program, *Report of the Expert Panel On Detection, Evaluation, and Treatment of High Blood*

Cholesterol in Adults, National Heart, Lung, and Blood Institute, National Institutes of Health, 1987.

12. Committee on Diet and Health, p. 13.
13. National Cancer Institute.
14. K. Carroll et al., "Fat and Cancer," *Cancer* 58 (1986): 1818–1825.
15. M. Enig, R. Munn, and M. Keeney, "Dietary Fat and Cancer Trends—A Critique," *Federation Proceedings* 37 (1978): 2215–2220.

CHAPTER 5

1. Charlotte Poleman and Christine Capra, *Shackelton's Nutrition Essentials and Diet Therapy* 5th ed. (Philadelphia: W. B. Saunders Co. (1984), 76.
2. U.S Department of Agriculture, "Nationwide Food Consumption Survey."
3. Nathan Smith, *Food For Sport* (Palo Alto, CA: Bull Publishing, 1976), 91.
4. B. Saltin, "Fluid, Electrolyte, and Energy Losses and Their Replenishment in Prolonged Exercise." In *Nutrition, Physical Fitness, and Health,* vol. 7, ed. J. Parizkova and V. A. Rogosksin (Baltimore: University Park Press, 1978).
5. L. Lefferts and S. Schmidt, "Water: Safe to Swallow?" *Nutrition Action* 15, no. 9 (1988): 1–7.
6. K. Cantor et al., "Bladder Cancer, Drinking Water Source, and Tap Water Consumption: A Case Control Study," *Journal of National Cancer Institute* 79, no. 6 (1987): 1269–1279.
7. "Bottled Waters Making Big Splash With More Than 700 Brands," *Environmental Nutrition* 11, no. 5 (1988): 4–5.
8. A. Schepers, "Drinking Water: Guarding Against Impurities," *Environmental Nutrition* 12, no. 9 (1989): 1.
9. "Thirsty or Not—Drink More Fluids," *Tufts University Diet and Nutrition Letter* 6, no. 5 (1988): 1–2.
10. Briggs and Calloway, p. 322.
11. Committee on Diet and Health, pp. 516–518.
12. National Cancer Institute.
13. U.S. Department of Agriculture, *Nationwide Food Consumption Survey. Continuing Survey of Food Intakes of Individuals. Women 19–50 Years and Their Children 1–5 Years, 4 Days, 1985,* Report No. 85-4 (Hyattsville, MD: Nutrition Monitoring Division, Human Nutrition Information Services, 1987).
14. Chenault, pp. 382–383.

15. National Heart, Lung, and Blood Institute, *Kit '89: Ideas and Materials for Preventing Heart Disease, Lung Disease, and Stroke,* U.S. Department of Health and Human Services, Public Health Service, National Institutes of Health, 1989.
16. "Is It Necessary to Cut Down on Salt After All?" *Tufts University Diet and Nutrition Letter* 6, no. 6 (1988): 1.
17. Committee on Diet and Health, pp. 41–84.

CHAPTER 6

1. S. Zeisel and J. Growden, "Diet and Brain Neurotransmitters," *Nutrition and the M.D.* 6 (1980): 1.
2. Eleanor Hamilton and Eva May Whitney, *Understanding Nutrition* 3rd ed. (St. Paul, MN: West Publishing, 1984), 561–562.
3. Committee on Diet and Health, p. 76.
4. Brody, p. 468.
5. National Cancer Institute.
6. Committee on Diet and Health, pp. 509–512.
7. Committee on Diet and Health, pp. 516–518.
8. Committee on Diet and Health, p. 519.
9. B. Worthington-Roberts and M. Breskin, "Supplementation Patterns of Washington State Dietitians," *Journal of American Dietetic Association* 84 (1984): 795.
10. H. A. Guthrie, "Supplementation: A Nutritionist's View," *Journal of Nutrition Education* 18 (1986): 130–132.
11. K. Helzlsouer, R. Jacobs, and S. Morris, "Acute Selenium Intoxication in the United States," *Federal Proceedings* 44 (1985): 1670.

Resources

BOOKS

Bailey, Covert. *Fit or Fat?* Boston: Houghton Mifflin Co., 1978.

Easy to read, this book makes important points about exercise and diet. It is a good "starter" book for those interested in exercise or weight management and explains the difference between losing weight and losing fat.

Bennett, William, M.D., and Joel Gurin. *The Dieter's Dilemma: The Setpoint Theory of Weight Control.* New York: Harper & Row Publishers, Basic Books, 1983.

The average weight of Americans keeps increasing despite our fondness for reducing diets. Two distinguished science writers point to overwhelming evidence that diets do not result in permanent weight loss. They discuss accumulating evidence that, for most people, weight is physiologically regulated around a setpoint that dieting cannot alter. The importance of physical activity in long-term weight management is discussed.

Bock, Allan S., M.D. *Food Allergies: A Primer for People.* New York: Vantage, 1988.

Dr. Bock does a good job of simplifying the complexities of food allergies and presenting scientific, well-documented facts about this subject. He exposes many fads and fallacies and offers guidelines for testing.

Brody, Jane. *Jane Brody's Nutrition Book.* New York: Bantam Books, 1987.

This comprehensive book covers topics ranging from an explanation of essential nutrients, to concerns about caffeine, to understanding food labels. It covers the special needs of various groups including pregnant women, babies, children, adolescents, vegetarians, athletes, and the elderly. Brody's weight control section examines the causes of obesity, the dangers of fad diets, and offers a lifelong, sensible approach to eating well. A useful book.

Brody, Jane. *Jane Brody's Good Food Book: Living the High Carbohydrate Way.* New York: W. W. Norton & Co., 1985.

This book shows how to plan a high-carbohydrate diet. The chapters are organized by major starches such as potatoes, beans, pasta, fruits, vegetables, nuts, and seeds. The chapter on

weight control provides guidelines on how to establish eating and exercise habits to achieve and maintain a normal body weight without dieting. The second half is a cookbook with over 350 recipes and menus.

Clark, Nancy. *Nancy Clark's Sports Nutrition Guide: Eating to Fuel Your Active Lifestyle.* Champaign, IL: Human Kinetics, Leisure Print, 1990.

This book shows how to create a diet for lifelong health. Clark shares examples of the nutrition advice she's given to all types of athletes, from weekend exercisers to Olympic athletes. She provides many how-to food suggestions and 103 fast, practical, and nutritious recipes appropriate for sports diets.

Coleman, Ellen. *Eating for Endurance.* Palo Alto, CA: Bull Publishing, 1988.

This informative book explains many aspects of exercise physiology, how oxygen and fuel affect athletic performance, and how to train, pace, eat, and drink to get optimum results. Topics included are carbohydrates, hydration, the use and abuse of sugar, and optimum pacing for training and performance. There are also chapters on common misconceptions about fasting, protein, fad diets, and weight loss.

Connor, Sonja L., and William E. Connor, M.D. *The New American Diet.* New York: Simon & Schuster, 1986.

The program presented in this book is divided into three phases geared to ease the reader into life-style changes, especially in the area of lowering fat intake. Phase one covers modifying existing habits and recipes. Phase two presents new recipes and steps to reduce meat intake. Phase three places emphasis on beans and grains as the primary protein sources, with fat intake reduced to 20 percent and carbohydrate intake increased to 65 percent of one's total daily nutrients. This book is useful in developing a diet to prevent major diseases such as heart disease, high blood pressure, stroke, and cancer.

Cooper, Kenneth, M.D. *Controlling Cholesterol: Dr. Kenneth H. Cooper's Preventive Medicine Program.* New York: Bantam Books, 1988.

This book offers a step-by-step program for assessing and controlling cholesterol levels and

168

reducing the risk of cardiovascular disease. Cooper covers the effects on your heart of coffee, alcohol, oat bran, fiber, fish oils, olive oil, birth control pills, smoking, and stress. He explains how to obtain an accurate lipid profile for blood fats and how to implement the right exercise program to control coronary disease.

Franz, Marion J. *Fast Food Facts*. South Bend, IN: Diamond Communications, 1990.

This book covers food items from 26 fast-food restaurant chains. Included are tables of calories, carbohydrates, protein, fat, and sodium, plus advice on which items should be avoided by diabetics.

Gershoff, Stanley, Ph.D. *The Tufts University Guide to Total Nutrition*. New York: Harper & Row, 1990.

This comprehensive and up-to-date volume by the dean of the prestigious Tufts University School of Nutrition is written in a style that makes it particularly easy to read and use. An introductory section on nutrition fundamentals is followed by sections that deal with the American diet, nutritional life-cycles, the diet-health connection, and keeping fit and trim. Based on the latest research findings, it features a series of nutrition quizzes and contains many practical suggestions for better eating.

Goor, Ron, M.D., and Nancy Goor. *Eater's Choice: A Food Lover's Guide to Lower Cholesterol*. Boston: Houghton Mifflin Co., 1987.

Reducing and controlling blood cholesterol can be accomplished by making food choices that both lower blood cholesterol and taste good. This book covers important information about diet and heart disease, clarifies the key relationship between saturated fat and risk of heart attack, and provides two weeks of meal plans and more than 200 recipes.

Gussow, Joan Dye. *The Feeding Web: Issues in Nutritional Ecology*. Palo Alto, CA: Bull Publishing, 1978.

In this book about food and the environment, a nationally known nutritionist explores the many links between the growing, distribution, and marketing of food, the health of societies, and the state of the physical environment. The book is a compilation of thoughtful articles written by people involved in various fields, such as nutrition, agriculture, and economics, providing insights into the relationship of American eating habits to world food problems.

Lappé, Frances M. *Diet for a Small Planet*. New York: Ballantine Books, 1982.

This is a handbook of vegetarian diets, protein myths, agricultural practices and their effect on world hunger, as well as a cookbook. The author explores the hidden costs of animal food production, the health problems of the current American diet, and how eating habits in industrialized countries affect developing nations. The many recipes show how to provide adequate protein in the diet without meat, poultry, or fish. Numerous charts, tables, and resource lists provide additional information.

Mond, Arlene, and Marion J. Franz. *Convenience Food Facts*. Minnetonka, MN: Diabetes Center, 1987.

This book contains information on more than 1,500 popular name-brand processed foods from 75 companies. The nutrition tables contain information on the calories, carbohydrates, protein, fat, and sodium content of each food, plus exchange values for diabetics. Warnings about products that are high in sugar, salt, or fat are also included.

Robertson, Laurel, Carol Flinders, and Brian Ruppenthal. *The New Laurel's Kitchen*. Berkeley: Ten Speed Press, 1986.

Recipes in this new edition of a classic vegetarian nutrition book have been revised to lower fat content and enhance health. Tables show the nutrient composition of foods used in each recipe. The nutrition section of the book contains over 100 pages of material based on current research about vegetarian eating habits.

Roth, Geneen. *Breaking Free From Compulsive Eating*. New York: Macmillan, 1985.

This book reveals the struggles and anxieties the author experienced being both overweight and anorexic, and relates her success in overcoming "a hunger that goes deeper than a need for food." She shares her learning experiences from therapy, workshops, lectures, and relationships.

Sacker, Ira M., M.D., and Marc A. Zimmer. *Dying to Be Thin: Understanding and Defeating Anorexia Nervosa and Bulimia—A Practical, Lifesaving Guide*. New York: Warner Books, 1987.

Two eating disorder therapists explain in detail the causes and symptoms of these disorders and where to find help. They include case histories of patients, families, and friends and show how to stop focusing on food and overcome anorexia and bulimia.

Tribole, Evelyn. *Eating on the Run*. Champaign, IL: Human Kinetics, Leisure Print, 1987.

If you live in the fast lane, this book can help you combine nutritious eating with your lifestyle. Included are 24 recipes for dishes that can be prepared in less than one minute, advice on dining out, eating fast foods and convenience foods, planning meals and snacks, and using calorie and nutrition charts to guide your eating selections.

Yetiv, Jack Z., M.D. *Popular Nutritional Practices: Sense and Nonsense*. Toledo: Popular Medicine Press, 1988.

Every day new nutritional facts make headlines. Using data compiled over 5 years of research, Yetiv offers facts about such issues as life extension, megavitamins, herbal remedies, food allergies, weight-loss diets, hypoglycemia, hair analysis, osteoporosis, and more.

NEWSLETTERS

Consumer Reports Health Letter is published monthly by Consumers Union, a nonprofit organization to provide information and advice on goods, services, health, and personal finance. A one-year subscription is $24 and may be obtained by calling (800) 274-8370.

Environmental Nutrition: The Professional Newsletter of Diet, Nutrition and Health is an interesting monthly publication featuring informative and reliable articles on diet and nutrition. A one-year subscription is $36 and may be obtained by writing to Environmental Nutrition, 2112 Broadway, New York, NY 10023.

Mayo Clinic Nutrition Letter is a monthly publication which provides reliable information about nutrition and fitness and how decisions on these matters affect your health. A one-year subscription is $24 and may be obtained by writing to Mayo Foundation for Medical Education and Research, 200 1st Street SW, Rochester, MN 55905, or calling (800) 888-3968.

Nutrition Action Health Letter is published 10 times a year by the Center for Science in the Public Interest. CSPI is a nonprofit public interest organization that advocates improved health and nutrition policies. This publication contains practical information on nutrition, food products,

and healthy recipes. Annual subscription cost is $19.95. You may write or call CSPI, 1501 16th Street, NW, Washington, DC 20036, or (202) 332-9110.

Running & FitNews is published monthly by the American Running and Fitness Association, a nonprofit educational association of athletes and sportmedicine professionals. This newsletter provides information on exercise guidelines, injuries, diet, and health-related fitness topics. A one-year subscription is $25 and may be obtained by writing to AR&FA, 9310 Old Georgetown Road, Bethesda, MD 20814, (301) 897-0197.

Tufts University Diet & Nutrition Letter is published monthly and covers a multitude of topics about diet and nutrition. A one-year subscription is $20 and may be obtained by writing to Tufts Diet & Nutrition Letter, P.O. Box 57857, Boulder, CO 80322-7857, (800) 274-7581. In Colorado, call (303) 447-9330.

University of California Berkeley Wellness Letter is published monthly and covers many topics, including nutrition, fitness, and stress management. A one-year subscription is $20 and may be obtained by writing to University of California, Berkeley Wellness Letter, P.O. Box 420148, Palm Coast, Florida 32142.

PERIODICALS

American Health Magazine: Fitness of Body and Mind is published 10 times a year and covers every aspect of physical and mental well-being. In addition to feature articles, ongoing departments include Nutrition News, Fitness Reports, Mind/Body News, Family Report, Family Pet and more. A one-year subscription is $14.95 and may be obtained by writing to American Health: Fitness of Body and Mind, P.O. Box 3015, Harlan, IA 51537-3015.

Cooking Light Magazine is published 6 times a year. Developed by nutritionists and dietitians, this colorful magazine is a wealth of information on cooking with less fat and sugar and contains interesting food and nutrition articles, practical meal-planning information, and creative recipes with amounts of fat, cholesterol, sodium, and calories per serving provided. A one-year subscription is $12 and is available from Cooking Light, P.O. Box C-549, Birmingham, AL 35283.

In Health Magazine is published 6 times a year and provides articles on a number of health issues, including nutrition. In addition to recipes and practical nutrition tips, the magazine regularly includes self-help resources for consumers. A one-year subscription is $18 and can be obtained by writing to In Health, P.O. Box 52431, Boulder, CO 80321-2431.

HOTLINES

American Diabetes Association, (800) ADA-DISC. Staff members will answer general questions about diabetes, risk factors, and symptoms. Free literature will be sent upon request and a free quarterly newsletter, *Diabetes '90*. Service available 8:30 A.M. to 5:00 P.M., Eastern Standard Time, Monday through Friday.

Bulimia Anorexia Self-Help, (800) 227-4785. Information is provided to callers about eating disorders and related problems, such as depression, phobias, and anxiety. Available 8:30 A.M. to 5:00 P.M., Monday through Friday, Central Standard Time. A crisis line is also available: Bulimia Anorexia Self-Help Crisis Line, (800) 762-3334, available 24 hours a day, 7 days a week.

Cancer Information Service, (800) 4-CANCER. This hotline is funded by the National Cancer Institute and staffed by professionals and volunteers. They will answer questions on causes of cancer, prevention, detection, and treatment and counsel about cancer-related problems. Literature is available and referrals are made to cancer support groups, treatment facilities, and transportation services. Available 9:00 A.M. to 10:00 P.M., Monday through Friday and 10:00 A.M. to 6:00 P.M. Saturday, Eastern Standard Time.

National Health Information Center, (800) 336-4797 (in Maryland, call (301) 656-4167). Operated by the Office of Disease Prevention and Health Promotion, this information and referral center's trained personnel will direct you to the national organization or government agency that can assist you with your health question, whether it's about high blood pressure, cancer, premenstrual syndrome, or any other topic. Available 9:00 A.M. to 5:00 P.M., Eastern Standard Time, Monday through Friday.

National Pesticide Telecommunications Network Hotline, (800) 858-PEST. Texas Tech University operates this service, funded by the Environmental Protection Agency. Health and environmental questions are answered about pesticides used around the house and garden and on supermarket fruits and vegetables. Available 24 hours a day, 7 days a week.

Safe Drinking Water Hotline, (800) 426-4791; (202) 382-5533 in Washington, DC. This hotline is funded by the Environmental Protection Agency and staffed by trained professionals who answer questions about water quality, water testing (what to test for and who can test your water), and regulations governing the water supply. They answer questions about bottled water and home water treatment as well. Available 8:30 A.M. to 4:30 P.M. Eastern Standard Time, Monday through Friday.

State list of Consulting Nutritionists. The American Dietetic Association will send you a list of consulting nutritionists in private practice in your state who can help you plan a healthier diet, lose weight, cope with high blood pressure, develop an optimal sports diet, or counsel you on any of a number of special nutritional needs. Nutritionists on the list are registered dietitians, meaning each is a nutrition expert with a degree in nutrition or a related science from an accredited institution, has passed a national certifying exam, and receives ongoing education in order to remain certified. Send a self-addressed stamped envelope to Nutrition Resources Department, American Dietetic Association, 216 W. Jackson Boulevard, Suite 800, Chicago, IL 60606-6995.

U.S. Department of Agriculture's Meat and Poultry Hotline, (800) 535-4555. Questions are answered about the proper handling, labeling, and safety of meat and poultry. They will also advise you on what to do if you find food you think may be unsafe. Available 10:00 A.M. to 4:00 P.M. Eastern Standard Time, Monday through Friday.

VIDEOTAPES

The College of Agriculture, University of Arizona, *Winning Sports Nutrition: The Competition Diet* (24 min., 1989).
The College of Agriculture, University of Arizona, *Winning Sports Nutrition: The Training Diet* (24 min., 1989).
These two programs feature nutrition experts plus high-profile athletes and coaches providing solid nutrition information and will inter-

est athletes, coaches, parents, and educators.
Leni Reed. *Lower Your Cholesterol, Now!* (58
min., 1989).

> This highly informative tape teaches you how
> to select foods to reduce cholesterol and fat in
> your diet. Reed presents specific ways to reduce
> one's intake of saturated fat as well as tips on
> cooking and food preparation.

Leni Reed. *Supermarket Savvy Tour Video.* (52
min., 1987).

> This video takes viewers on a tour through a
> supermarket, while Reed instructs in the art of
> reading labels. You will learn how to make
> informed, healthier choices of food and how to
> sort out the important information from the
> hype. A valuable resource for consumers con-
> cerned about lowering cholesterol and fat
> intake.

Art Ulene, M.D. *Count Out Cholesterol* (75 min.,
with booklet). New York: Random House, Inc.,
1989.

> This is a video version of Dr. Ulene's book
> *Count Out Cholesterol* and includes shopping
> and cooking tips, accurate advice on lowering
> cholesterol, and a demostration of the Rockport
> Fitness Walking Test. Available through book-
> stores or from Nutrition Counseling and Edu-
> cation Services, (800) 445-5653.

ADVOCACY AND CONSUMER GROUPS

American Diabetes Association, 2 Park Avenue
New York, NY 10016

> This organization advocates for the continuing
> research, education, and treatment of diabetes.
> Numerous educational materials useful to dia-
> betics are available. State and local chapters
> are excellent resources for information.

American Dietetic Association (Nutrition) (ADA),
216 W. Jackson Boulevard, Suite 800, Chicago, IL
60606, (312) 899-0040

> ADA is an organization of professionals in the
> practice of dietetics in hospitals, colleges, uni-
> versities, school food service, day care centers,
> research, business and industry. ADA provides
> direction and leadership for the practice of
> dietetics, education, and research and promotes
> optimal health and nutrition for the popula-
> tion. Publication: *Journal of the American Di-
> etetic Association* (monthly).

American Heart Association, 7320 Greenville Avenue Dallas, TX 75231

> An organization that disseminates extensive
> nutrition information aimed at preventing
> heart disease, publishes cookbooks, and offers
> public and worksite programs in heart health.
> State chapters are excellent information
> resources.

American Medical Association, Nutrition Information Section, 535 North Dearborn Street, Chicago, IL 60610

> The AMA disseminates scientific information
> to members and the public. Informs members
> on significant medical and health legislation
> on state and national levels and represents the
> profession before Congress and governmental
> agencies. Ad hoc committees are formed for
> such topics as health care planning and princi-
> ples of medical ethics.

Center for Science in the Public Interest (CSPI),
1755 S Street, NW, Washington, DC 20009

> CSPI monitors food manufacturers and federal
> agencies involved in food regulation, safety,
> and trade. They investigate and initiate legal
> action against unsafe and unfair practices re-
> lated to food and nutrition. They publish nutri-
> tion education materials and a newsletter
> covering nutrition and health, food regulation
> updates, and healthful cooking. Publication:
> *Nutrition Action* (monthly).

Community Nutrition Institute (CNI), 2001 S
Street, NW, Suite 530, Washington, DC 20009,
(202) 462-4700

> CNI advocates for food and nutrition issues
> which include hunger, food quality and safety,
> nutrition research, food programs, education,
> and food labeling and marketing. Their major
> goal is to secure a food system that sustains
> cultural and social values and maintains hu-
> man health. CNI assists federal agencies in
> analyzing and implementing food programs
> and research, in developing standards for food
> products, and lobbies for USDA and FDA rat-
> ification. Publication: *Nutrition Week* (weekly).

Society For Nutrition Education (SNE), 1700
Broadway, Suite 300, Oakland, CA 94612, (415)
444-7133

> SNE members are nutrition educators from the
> fields of dietetics, public health, home eco-
> nomics, medicine, industry, and education (ele-
> mentary, secondary, college, university, and
> consumer affairs). Their goal is to promote
> nutritional well-being for the North American
> public. SNE maintains, produces, and sells nu-
> trition education materials and films (in En-

glish and Spanish). Publication: *Journal of Nutrition Education* (bimonthly).

ORGANIZATIONS CONCERNED WITH HUNGER:

Bread for the World, 6411 Chillum Place, NW,Washington, DC 20012

This is an organization of Christian citizens with local chapters around the country. It works to influence legislation concerning hunger issues. Publications: newsletter and various reports.

Food Research and Action Center (FRAC), 2011 I Street, NW, Washington, DC 20006

This group advocates for public food programs that benefit the poor in the United States, and supports organizations of low-income people that defend needed programs.

Institute for Food and Development Policy, 1885 Mission Street, San Francisco, CA 94103

An organization that researches and publishes information on U.S. agricultural trade practices, alternative agricultural development in other countries, and economic and land use issues that contribute to hunger. Publications: *Food First News* (quarterly newsletter), *Action Alerts*, catalog of books and reports.

Interreligious Taskforce on U.S. Food Policy Meals for Millions/Freedom from Hunger Foundation, 1800 Olympic Boulevard, P.O. Drawer 680, Santa Monica, CA 90406

An organization that brings together various religious groups to influence U.S. policies that affect hunger abroad and at home. Publication: *Hunger* (4-6 issues/year).

Index

174

Page 3 © 1990, The American Dietetic Association. *ADA Courier,* vol. 29, no. 3. Used by permission. Page 5 Reprinted from *In Health.* Copyright © 1989. Page 12 Figure 1.3 Copyright 1981, CSPI. Reprinted from *Nutrition Action Healthletter* (1875 Connecticut Ave., NW, Suite 300, Washington, DC 20009-5728. $19.95 for 10 issues). Page 13 Copyright 1990, CSPI. Reprinted from *Nutrition Action Healthletter* (1875 Connecticut Ave., NW, Suite 300, Washington, DC 20009-5728. $19.95 for 10 issues). Page 16 Reprinted with permission from *Environmental Nutrition Newsletter,* 2112 Broadway #200, New York, NY 10023. Page 18 Reprinted by permission of the American Cancer Society, Inc. Page 24 Table 2.1 Reprinted from *Recommended Dietary Allowances* by permission. Page 30 Table 2.4 Copyright 1990, CSPI. Reprinted from *Nutrition Action Healthletter* (1875 Connecticut Ave., NW, Suite 300, Washington, DC 20009-5728. $19.95 for 10 issues). Page 32 Table 2.5 From *The Nutrition Desk Reference,* Copyright © 1985, 1990 by Robert H. Garrison, Jr., and Elizabeth Somer, published by Keats Publishing, Inc., New Canaan, CT. Used with permission. Page 33 Table 2.6 From *The Nutrition Desk Reference,* Copyright © 1985, 1990 by Robert H. Garrison, Jr., and Elizabeth Somer, published by Keats Publishing, Inc., New Canaan, CT. Used with permission. Page 35 Reprinted with permission from *Environmental Nutrition Newsletter,* 2112 Broadway #200, New York, NY 10023. Page 37 Reprinted with permission from *Environmental Nutrition Newsletter,* 2112 Broadway #200, New York, NY 10023. Page 39 Table 2.7 Reprinted by permission of *Redbook Magazine.* Copyright © 1989 by The Hearst Corporation. All rights reserved. Page 41 From *Tufts University Diet & Nutrition Letter,* April 1988, pp.

3-6. Reprinted by permission. Page 51 Table 3.1 From Metropolitan Life Insurance Company, Health and Safety Education Division. Page 52 From *Tufts University Diet & Nutrition Letter,* October 1989, pp. 3, 6. Reprinted by permission. Page 56 From *Tufts University Diet & Nutrition Letter,* December 1989, p. 2. Reprinted by permission. Page 58 From *Tufts University Diet & Nutrition Letter,* December 1989, pp. 1-2. Reprinted by permission. Page 59 Reprinted by permission of *University of California, Berkeley Wellness Letter,* © Health Letter Associates, 1989. Page 64 © 1987, The American Dietetic Association. *The Dietary Guidelines: Seven Ways to Help Yourself to Good Health and Nutrition.* Used by permission. Page 66 From *Nutrition and Health* by Alice A. Chenault, p. 49. Copyright © 1984 by Holt, Rinehart & Winston, Inc., reprinted by permission of the publisher. Page 68 Reprinted by permission of *University of California, Berkeley Wellness Letter,* © Health Letter Associates, 1989. Page 71 Table 3.4 Reprinted from "How Sweet Is It?" which is available from the Center for Science in the Public Interest, 1875 Connecticut Ave., NW, Suite 300, Washington, DC 20009-5728. Copyright © 1985. Page 74 From *Nutrition and Health* by Alice A. Chenault, p. 186. Copyright © 1984 by Holt, Rinehart & Winston, Inc., reprinted by permission of the publisher. Page 81 Reprinted with permission from *Environmental Nutrition Newsletter,* 2112 Broadway #200, New York, NY 10023. Page 85 Copyright © 1989 by The New York Times Company. Reprinted by permission. Page 89 From *Tufts University Diet & Nutrition Letter,* July 1988, pp. 3-6. Reprinted by permission. Page 100 Table 4.9 ©1987, The American Dietetic Association. *The Dietary Guidelines: Seven Ways to Help Yourself To Good Health and Nutri-*

tion. Used by permission. Page 101 From *The Johns Hopkins Medical Letter,* January 1990. © 1990 Medletter Associates, Inc. Page 104 Reprinted with permission from *Environmental Nutrition Newsletter,* 2112 Broadway #200, New York, NY 10023. Page 107 From *Tufts University Diet & Nutrition Letter,* July 1988, pp. 1-2. Reprinted by permission. Page 109 Reprinted permission of *University of California, Berkeley Wellness Letter,* ©Health Letter Associates, 1990. Page 112 Copyright 1988, CSPI. Reprinted from *Nutrition Action Healthletter* (1875 Connecticut Ave., NW, Suite 300, Washington, DC 20009-5728. $19.95 for 10 issues). Page 116 From *Tufts University Diet & Nutrition Letter,* June 1989, p. 1. Reprinted by permission. Page 129 Reprinted with permission from *Environmental Nutrition Newsletter,* 2112 Broadway #200, New York, NY 10023. Page 131 Figure 5.1 Reprinted with permission from *Environmental Nutrition Newsletter,* 2112 Broadway #200, New York, NY 10023. Page 135 Reprinted with permission from *Environmental Nutrition Newsletter,* 2112 Broadway #200, New York, NY 10023. Page 138 Reprinted with permission from *Environmental Nutrition Newsletter,* 2112 Broadway #200, New York, NY 10023. Page 142 Figure 6.1 Courtesy of Stouffer Foods Corporation. Page 144 Reprinted permission of *University of California, Berkeley Wellness Letter,* ©Health Letter Associates, 1990. Page 147 Reprinted with permission from *Environmental Nutrition Newsletter,* 2112 Broadway #200, New York, NY 10023. Page 151 Reprinted with permission from *Environmental Nutrition Newsletter,* 2112 Broadway #200, New York, NY 10023. Page 153 Reprinted with permission from *Environmental Nutrition Newsletter,* 2112 Broadway #200, New York, NY 10023.